前 言

　　2012 年欧洲心脏病学会（European Society of Cardiology，ESC）发表上一版指南 5 年以来，ST 段抬高型心肌梗死（ST-elevation myocardial infarction，STEMI）领域的争议主要集中在战术层面。然而，一个严酷的事实是，尽管做出了很大的努力，但是 STEMI 患者的死亡率仍然很高，尤其是存活患者的心力衰竭发生率更高，因此，有必要从战略层面更新 STEMI 的救治概念和体系。2017 年 8 月 25 日适时发表的新版 STEMI 指南体现了提高再灌注治疗率和降低死亡率这样一个 STEMI 救治的精髓，非常值得借鉴。

　　虽然新版 STEMI 指南力求体现提高再灌注治疗率和降低死亡率这样一个核心理念，值得借鉴，然而，欧美资料显示，心肌梗死存活患者的 5 年死亡率为 10%，心力衰竭发生率更是达到 70% 以上。因此，如何全面有效地保护心肌，降低心力衰竭发生率是救治 STEMI 患者的另一个大目标。遗憾的是，新版指南在此方面涉及太少，期待在下一版指南中有所体现。

　　为了帮助中国同行进一步理解 ESC 新版指南，我们在编译该指南的基础上，在每一章后进行评注，编写了这本《解读欧洲急性心肌梗死治疗指南.2018》，供同道们参考。

　　本书的出版得到了中国医学科学院医学与健康科技创新工程基金（2016-I2M-1-009）的支持。

颜红兵　赵汉军

2018 年 1 月 1 日于国家心血管病中心

目 录

第一章　序 1
　　评　注 3

第二章　引　言 6
　　第 1 节　急性心肌梗死的定义 6
　　第 2 节　ST 段抬高型心肌梗死流行病学 7
　　评　注 8

第三章　2017 年版新在哪儿? 10

第四章　紧急处理 11
　　第 1 节　初步诊断 11
　　第 2 节　减轻疼痛、呼吸困难和焦虑 15
　　第 3 节　心脏骤停 16
　　第 4 节　院前治疗后勤保障 18
　　评　注 23

第五章　再灌注治疗 25
　　第 1 节　再灌注策略的选择 25
　　第 2 节　直接经皮冠状动脉介入治疗和辅助治疗 29
　　第 3 节　溶栓和药物有创策略 39
　　第 4 节　外科冠状动脉旁路移植术 45
　　评　注 46

第六章　住院期间和出院时的处理 64
　　第 1 节　冠状动脉监护病房 / 重症监护病房 64
　　第 2 节　监护 64
　　第 3 节　离床活动 65

第 4 节　住院时间 65

第 5 节　特殊患者 66

第 6 节　风险评估 72

评　注 75

第七章　ST 段抬高型心肌梗死的长期治疗 77

第 1 节　生活方式干预和危险因素控制 77

第 2 节　抗栓治疗 80

第 3 节　β - 受体阻滞剂 84

第 4 节　降脂治疗 87

第 5 节　硝酸酯类 89

第 6 节　钙拮抗药 89

第 7 节　血管紧张素转换酶抑制剂和血管紧张素 Ⅱ 受体阻滞剂 89

第 8 节　盐皮质激素和醛固酮受体拮抗剂 90

评　注 93

第八章　ST 段抬高型心肌梗死的并发症 95

第 1 节　心肌功能紊乱 95

第 2 节　心力衰竭 97

第 3 节　急性期心律失常和传导异常的处理 102

第 4 节　机械性并发症 107

第 5 节　心包炎 108

评　注 109

第九章　无冠状动脉阻塞的心肌梗死 111

评　注 113

第十章　医疗质量评估 114

评　注 117

第十一章　缺乏证据和将来研究的领域 118

第十二章　本指南要点 121

第十三章　重要建议小结 125

参考文献 129

第一章 ⊕ 序

　　指南总结和评估现有的证据，旨在帮助医务人员为某种情况下的具体患者选择最佳的治疗策略。指南及其相关建议应当帮助医务人员在其日常实践中做出决策。然而，对某一个具体患者的最终决策，应当由其经治医务人员与患者本人和照顾患者的相关人员共同做出。

　　近年来，欧洲心脏病学会（European Society of Cardiology，ESC）及其他学会和组织，已经发布了大量的指南和重点更新。鉴于对临床实践的影响，为了使所有决策透明化，已经建立了制订指南的质量标准。可以在 ESC 网站上查询到制订和发布 ESC 指南的相关建议（http://www.escardio.org/Guidelines-&-Education/Clinical-Practice-Guidelines/Guidelines-development/Writing-ESC-Guidelines）。ESC 指南代表了 ESC 就某一问题的官方立场，并且会定期更新。

　　由 ESC 挑选的本工作组成员，包括来自 ESC 相关亚专业，以代表涉及本病患者医疗的专业人员。经过挑选的本领域的专家，根据 ESC 实用指南委员会的政策，全面审核了有关处理某一种疾病已经发表的证据。对诊断性和治疗性操作进行严格的评估，包括评估风险 - 获益比。根据预先定义，对某一个处理的证据水平和建议力度进行权衡和分级（表 1-1 和表 1-2）。

　　编写组和审核组的专家要提供所有可能被认为是实际或潜在利益冲突来源关系的申报表。将这些申报表编辑归档，并且可以在 ESC 网站查询（http://www.escardio.org/guidelines）。在编写过程中新出现的利益冲突，将告知 ESC 并且进行更新。工作

表 1-1　建议分类

建议分类	定义	建议用词
Ⅰ类	证据表明和（或）共识认为某种治疗或操作有益、有用或有效	建议
Ⅱ类	某种治疗或操作的用途或效果的证据有矛盾和（或）意见有分歧	
Ⅱa类	证据或意见倾向于有用或有效	应当考虑
Ⅱb类	关于有用或有效的证据或意见不充分	可以考虑
Ⅲ类	证据表明和（或）共识认为某种治疗或操作无用或无效，并且在某些情况下可能有害	建议

表 1-2　证据水平

证据水平 A	数据来源于多个随机临床试验或荟萃分析
证据水平 B	数据来源于单个随机临床试验或大规模非随机试验
证据水平 C	专家共识和（或）数据来源于小规模研究、回顾性研究、注册研究

组的全部财政支持来自 ESC，没有医疗保健行业参与。

ESC 实用指南委员会监督和协调新指南的准备工作。该委员会还负责这些文件的背书过程。这些实用指南委员会的文件得到实用指南委员会和外部专家的广泛审查。经适当修订后，这些实用指南委员会的文件得到工作组所有专家的批准。最终文件由实用指南委员会批准在《欧洲心脏杂志》和《欧洲心胸外科杂志》上发表。从科学和医学知识及现有证据角度，进行认真审核后制订这些指南委员会文件。

制订 ESC 指南的任务还包括创建教育工具和对建议的实施计划，包括浓缩袖珍指南版本、摘要幻灯片、为非专业人员提供必要信息的小册子、数字应用电子版（智能手机等）及其他根据不同主题的教育工具。这些版本经过删减，因此，如果需要，应当参阅全文版，这些可以在 ESC 网站和《欧洲心脏杂志》网站免费获得。鼓励 ESC 的各个国家学会认可、翻译和实施所有 ESC 指南。实施方案是必要的，因为已经表明，疾病的结果可能受到完全应用临床建议的有利影响。

需要调查和注册登记来验证日常实践并且与指南的建议保持一致，从而完成从临床研究到指南编写、再到正式重点更新和进行宣传并且在临床实践中实施这个循环过程。

鼓励医务人员应用 ESC 指南时全面进行临床判断，以及制订和实施预防、诊断或治疗策略。然而，ESC 指南并不影响任何医疗专业人员在考虑具体患者的健康状况并且与患者本人或照顾患者的人员进行必要的讨论后个人作出的适当和准确的决策。医务人员也有责任在处方时核查有关药品和器械使用的规章制度。

⊕ | 评 注

由专业学会制订心血管疾病临床实用指南开始于美国，之后，包括中国在内的各个国家的专业学会也先后开始效仿，制订自己的指南，以指导本国实践。今天，美国心脏病学会（American College of Cardiology，ACC）和美国心脏协会（American Heart Association，AHA）及 ESC 制订的各个临床实用指南已经成为各国心血管医师的重要参考工具。美国 30 多年来的实践证明，临床实用指南对临床实践的影响力在不断扩大。虽然很难评估这些指南对临床实践的影响结果，但是 2012 年对 ACC 和 AHA 会员的调查显示，临床实践中常规应用指南率高达 90% 以上。

指导临床实践需要有高质量指南，而制订高质量指南必须有一个严密和复杂的科学程序，ACC 和 AHA 堪称是这方面的典范，值得国内借鉴。ACC 和 AHA 制订指南大体需要经历如下 6 个阶段：

（1）**组成团队** 由 ACC 和 AHA 来选择指南的主题并邀请相关学会参与。推选编委会主席并组成编写组，审查参与人员是否与相关企业有利益关系。召集编写组成员，提出指南编写大纲并分配任务。

（2）**提出问题** 由编写组和证据审核组先提出指南所涉及的相关问题，包括人群、干预、比较、结果、时机和背景。经过学会领导层和参与学会审核这些问题后，由编写组和证据审核组进行充实和修订，最后形成指南最终要涉及的问题。

（3）**审核证据** 由编写组和证据审核组分头完成。编写组负责检索文献，分析证据和选择相关文献，最后由编写组、相关人员和检索机构共同将证据编辑成表。与此同时，证据审核组与证据检索机构制订检索方案，由证据检索组两次筛选文章题目和摘要，并且两次筛选正文。根据证据表将所选文章进行数字化处理后，由证据审核组进行分析，写出全面综述。

（4）**形成初稿** 写作组提出指南建议，补充文献，并进行多次电话会议进行讨论。在全体会议上由编写组提出最终建议，更新正文，达成共识，在全体会议上根据编写组的讨论结果，进行最终修改。

（5）**专业评审** 交同行评审，并根据评审意见，修改初稿和修订建议。经指南工作组评审后，再经学会领导层批准，进入下一程序。

（6）**编辑出版** 经过编辑整理后，在线发表指南稿。经过排版和再次校对后，出版最终指南和系统综述，同时出版指南口袋本和幻灯片等。

为了展示指南中相关建议的强度和支持提出这些建议的循证学证据的质量，ACC和AHA建立了一套完整的标准。根据2015年8月ACC和AHA的最新修改意见，对指南中相关建议的强度分为3类5种情况，对循证学证据的级别也分为3个级别和5种情况：

（1）**建议分类及其含义** Ⅰ类建议的力度最强，获益远远大于风险。Ⅱa类建议力度次之，获益大于风险，而Ⅱb类建议力度较弱，获益稍大于风险。Ⅲ类建议分2种情况，一种是无获益，获益与风险相当，另一种是有害，风险大于获益。

（2）**证据分级及其含义** A级证据是来自3种情况的循证学证据：来自1个以上临床随机研究的高质量数据；来自对高质量临床随机研究的荟萃分析；得到高质量注册研究证实的1个或多个临床随机研究。B-R级证据来自2种情况：来自1个或多个临床随机研究、质量中等的数据；来自对中等质量临床随机研究的荟萃分析。B-NR级证据也来自2种情况：质量中等，来自1个或多个设计良好的非随机观察性或注册研究；对上述研究的荟萃分析。C-LD级证据来自3种情况：来自随机或非随机观察性或注册研究，有设计缺陷；对上述研究的荟萃分析；在人体进行的生理学和器械研究。C-LO级证据来自根据临床经验提出的专家共识。

虽然提倡指南指导实践，但是在实际应用中要注意 2 个问题。第一个问题是，欧美指南分别是根据欧洲人群和北美地区人群的临床实践而制订，不一定适合中国人群。一个典型的例子是目前欧美指南均不建议在急性心肌梗死患者直接经皮冠状动脉介入治疗时常规应用血栓抽吸术，而在中国血栓抽吸术的比例实际上很高。欧美患者与中国患者的不同表现在，欧美绝大多数患者在发病后 3 小时内接受再灌注治疗，而中国患者往往是在 6 小时之后才接受再灌注治疗，这可能部分解释了在发病 3 小时内冠状动脉内新鲜血栓的患者应用血栓抽吸效果不好的原因。第二个问题是，由于制订指南耗时，因此所参考的文献相对"过时"。例如，2015 年 ACC/AHA 急性心肌梗死直接经皮冠状动脉介入指南更新于 2015 年 10 月在线发表，2016 年 3 月正式发表，但是参考的文献全部发表在 2015 年 8 月以前。这个指南更新建议对于急性心肌梗死合并多支病变并且血流动力学稳定的患者，可以考虑对非梗死相关动脉采取一次性介入治疗。然而，多数专家认为，对于合并多支病变的患者，采用一次性策略还是分次策略更好，目前并无定论。实际上，与一次性策略比较，分次策略能够改善患者的早期和晚期存活。总之，在借鉴指南时，要清楚指南的产生背景，理解指南建议的力度和循证学证据的质量，认识指南没有或还不能回答的问题，结合患者的具体情况，更好地指导临床实践。

第二章
引 言

应当依据高质量临床试验所获得的可靠证据，并参考资深专家的意见，更新对 ST 段抬高型心肌梗死（ST-segment elevation myocardial infarction，STEMI）患者的处理。必须承认，即便是非常出色的临床试验，对其结果的解释也应当持开放态度，并且应当根据具体临床和资源情况调整治疗。

本指南工作组已尽最大努力与其他 ESC 指南和共识文件保持统一，包括同期发表的双联抗血小板治疗（dual antiplatelet therapy，DAPT）指南更新，力求与 ESC 指南策略保持一致。如表 1-1 和表 1-2 所列，依据已有的标准对某种治疗处理方案的证据水平和建议强度进行权衡和分级。即便建议的证据水平是基于专家的意见，本工作组决定也要为读者提供文献，供其在有些情况做决策时参考。

第 1 节　急性心肌梗死的定义

在心肌缺血的临床背景下存在心肌损伤坏死的证据（心脏肌钙蛋白值升高至少 1 次超过参考上限的第 99 百分位）时，可以定义为急性心肌梗死。日常实践中，为了迅速开始治疗（如再灌注治疗），当患者有持续性胸部不适或其他提示缺血的症状，同时至少 2 个相邻导联有 ST 段抬高时定义为 STEMI。相反，患者就诊时没有 ST 段抬高的情况通常定义为非 ST 段抬高型心肌梗死（non-ST-segment elevation myocardial infarction，NSTEMI），近期已经发表了 NSTEMI 指南。有些患者心肌梗死会形成 Q 波（Q 波心肌梗死），但多数患者并无 Q 波形成（非 Q 波心肌梗死）。

此外，根据心肌梗死的病理、临床、预后和治疗策略差异，可以将其分为不同类型（参考第 3 版全球心肌梗死定义，拟于 2018 年更新）。大多数 STEMI 患者属于 1 型心肌梗死（有冠状动脉血栓的证据），其余 STEMI 则属于其他类型心肌梗死。即使冠状动脉造影表现为非阻塞性冠状动脉疾病，也可以发生心肌梗死，包括 STEMI。这种类型的心肌梗死称为"非阻塞性冠状动脉心肌梗死（myocardial infarction with non-obstructive coronary arteries，MINOCA），将在第九章讨论。

第 2 节　ST 段抬高型心肌梗死流行病学

在世界范围内，缺血性心脏病是最常见的死因，其发病率还在不断增加。然而，过去三十年欧洲的缺血性心脏病死亡率有总体下降的趋势。尽管不同国家之间有较大差异，缺血性心脏病在欧洲每年导致近 180 万人死亡，或者占全因死亡的 20%。

STEMI 和 NSTEMI 的相对发病率分别呈下降和增加趋势。在瑞典设立的可能是最为全面的欧洲 STEMI 注册显示，2015 年 STEMI 的发病率为 58/100 000。其他欧洲国家 STEMI 的发病率为（43 ～ 144）/100 000。同样，在美国，STEMI 的校正发病率从 1999 年的 133/100 000 下降到 2008 年的 50/100 000，而 NSTEMI 的发病率则没有变化或略有增加。STEMI 年轻人比老年人多见，男性比女性多见。

STEMI 患者的死亡率受多种因素的影响，包括高龄、killip 分级、治疗延迟、是否有 STEMI- 医疗急救系统（emergency medical system，EMS）网络、治疗策略、既往心肌梗死史、糖尿病、肾衰竭、冠状动脉病变支数和左心室射血分数（left ventricular ejection fraction，LVEF）。近期几项研究显示，随着再灌注治疗、直接经皮冠状动脉介入治疗（primary percutaneous coronary intervention，PPCI）、现代抗栓治疗和二级预防的推广，STEMI 急性期和远期死亡率已有下降。然而，死亡率依然很高。ESC 成员国的国家注册数据显示，未经选择的 STEMI 患者住院死亡率为 4%～12%，而冠状动脉造影注册数据显示 STEMI 患者的年死亡率大约为 10%。

尽管女性缺血性心脏病发病比男性平均晚 7～10 年，心肌梗死仍然是女性死亡的首位病因。60 岁以下的人群中，男性急性冠状动脉综合征（acute coronary syndrome，ACS）发病率是女性的 3～4 倍，但是在 75 岁以上 ACS 人群中，女性患者占多数。女性心肌梗死的症状常常不典型，一些注册数据显示不典型症状可占 30%，就诊时间也有晚于男性的倾向。因此，女性有可疑缺血症状时，要对心肌梗死保持高度警惕。女性 PCI 出血并发症的风险也高。女性心肌梗死的预后是否更差尚在争议之中。一些研究提示，老龄和合并症多的女性心肌梗死患者预后更差。女性接受介入治疗和再灌注治疗的比例低于男性。本指南强调，女性和男性同样能从再灌注治疗和 STEMI 相关的治疗措施中获益，女性和男性的处理模式也不应有差别。

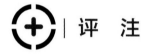

评 注

本章讨论了急性心肌梗死的定义和 STEMI 流行病学变化。

缺血性心脏病仍然是全世界最常见的死因之一。尽管 STEMI 和 NSTEMI 的相对发生率分别在下降和上升，并且与 STEMI 相关的急性和长期死亡率下降，但在广泛使用再灌注治疗的同时，死亡率仍然很高，欧洲 STEMI 患者的住院死亡率在 4%～12%。

临床诊断急性心肌梗死主要依据患者的临床表现、心电图表现和肌钙蛋白的检测结果。然而，临床实践中，相当多的患者并非表现"典型"，结果临床医师（尤其是年轻医师）不能及时做出诊断。实际上，"心绞痛"是一个不准确的翻译术语，原意是胸前区的一种压迫性的沉重感，因此，使用"闷"来描述比使用"痛"更准确。临床实践中，STEMI 患者表现为典型心绞痛者仅有 50%～75%，因此，临床面临的挑战是如何识别那些 25%～50% 表现不典型的患者，尤其是老年、合并糖尿病、肾功能不全和呼吸系统疾病的患者。判读心电图结果时一定要有不同时间的心电图比较。通常左回旋支闭塞的患者心电图变化快，表现为 ST 段抬高的时间窗短。因此在临床表现典型并且肌钙蛋白检测高值的患者，应当首先考虑左回旋支闭塞。冠状动脉三支病变发生 STEMI 的患者也可以 ST 段抬高的时间窗短，临床判读心电图时要考虑这种因素。肌钙蛋白（尤其是高敏肌钙蛋白）对于及时诊断心肌梗死至关重要，基线肌钙蛋白水平越高，患者的风险越高。然而，肌钙蛋白轻度增高（即使较正常上线值增高 10 倍以上），而患者临床表现并不十分典型，心电图 ST 段仅轻度增高，往往会给临床决策带来困惑。

急性心肌梗死在我国是一个更为严重的问题。与欧美国家不同，近 10 年来，中国急性心肌梗死发病率无论是在城市还是在农村均呈增高趋势，死亡率没有降低。由于没有广泛应用高敏肌钙蛋白和临床医师的认识受限导致漏诊，相信中国急性心肌梗死的实际发病率更高。

与欧美国家不同，中国 STEMI 的发生率并没有明显降低，但是在 ACS 患者中所占的比例有所下降。回顾性分析中国医学科学院阜外医院 2010—2017 年接受急诊 PCI 患者的资料显示，STEMI 在 ACS 患者中所占比例由 88.6% 降低到 73.5%，而非 ST 段抬高型急性冠状动脉综合征（NSTE-ACS）由 11.4% 增高到 26.5%。有关 STEMI 患者的死亡率，还缺乏全国性的资料。由于国内很多中心对于 STEMI 合并心源性休克的急诊介入治疗并不积极，因此无法得到有关 STEMI 急诊介入治疗患者死亡率的数据。

最后，尽管获益相同，但是女性比男性较少或延迟接受再灌注治疗和其他循证学治疗。在中国同样存在着女性患者较少或延迟接受循证学治疗，主要原因是女性患者的临床表现相对不典型，临床医师担心抗栓治疗和有创性检查、治疗带来的相关并发症。因此，要重视女性患者，提高这些患者接受再灌注治疗和其他循证学治疗的比例，改善临床预后。

第三章

2017 年版新在哪儿？

2017 年 STEMI 指南的创新点见图 3-1。

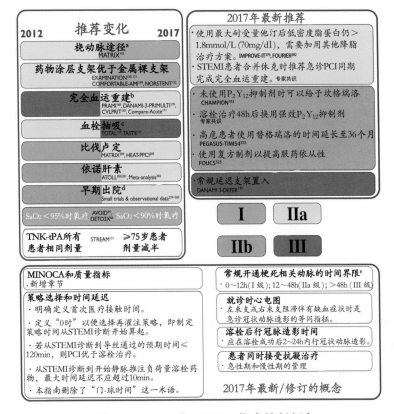

图 3-1 2017 年 STEMI 指南的创新点

注：PCI：经皮冠脉介入治疗；SaO₂：动脉血氧饱和度；STEMI：ST 段抬高型心肌梗死；TNK-tPA：替奈普酶组织型纤溶酶原激活剂。临床试验名字的释义参见相关列表。

ª只针对有经验的桡动脉路径术者。ᵇ出院前（可以是即刻也可以分次进行）。ᶜ常规血栓抽吸（在一些病例作为补救措施时可以考虑使用）。ᵈ2012 版指南定义早期出院为 72h 后；2017 版指南则定义为 48h～72h。ᵉ如果仍有症状或血流动力学不稳定，不论发病时间长短都应该开通梗死相关动脉。

第四章 ⊕
紧急处理

第1节　初步诊断

STEMI 的处理包括诊断和治疗，应当在首次医疗接触（first medical contact, FMC）时启动（表4-1）。建议建立区域性再灌注策略并使其发挥最大效益。

表4-1　初诊建议

建议	建议类别	证据水平
心电图监测		
首次医疗接触后尽快记录 12 导联 ECG 检查并判读，最迟不超过 10min	I	B
对所有疑诊 STEMI 的患者尽快心电除颤监护仪进行监测	I	B
高度怀疑后壁心肌梗死（回旋支闭塞）的患者应该考虑加做后壁导联心电图（$V_7 \sim V_9$）	II a	B
下壁心肌梗死患者应该考虑加做右室导联（V_3R 和 V_4R）心电图以明确是否合并右室心肌梗死	II a	B
血标本留取		
心肌梗死急性期尽早常规留取血进行血清标志物监测，但不能因此延迟再灌注治疗	I	C

首先必须做出 STEMI 的诊断。通常依据缺血的症状（持续胸痛）和体征（12 导联心电图）诊断 STEMI。这通常基于持续心肌缺血的症状（即持续胸痛）和 12 导联心电图检查。有冠心病史和放射至颈部、下颌、左臂的疼痛是心肌梗死的重要线索。部分患者表现不典型，如表现为气短、恶心或呕吐、乏力、心悸或晕厥。服用硝酸甘油（三硝酸甘油酯）后胸痛减轻可能会产生误导，不建议作为诊断依据。服用硝酸甘油后症状缓解时，必须再次获得 12 导联心电图。服用硝酸甘油后 ST 段完全回落并且症状完全缓解，提示冠状动脉痉挛（伴有或不伴有心肌梗死），建议早期做冠状动脉造影（24 小时内）。对于再发 ST 段抬高或胸痛的患者，应当立即进行冠状动脉造影。

建议对所有疑诊 STEMI 的患者尽快启动心电监测，以便发现危及生命的心律失常，必要时迅速电除颤。疑诊 STEMI 的患者必须在 FMC 时尽快获得并判读 12 导联心电图，加速 STEMI 的早期诊断和分诊。

对于临床怀疑心肌缺血并有 ST 段抬高的患者，需尽快启动再灌注治疗。心电图表现不确定或没有证据支持心肌梗死的怀疑诊断时，应重复心电图检查，尽可能与以往心电图记录进行对比。如果现场对院前心电图不能进行判读，建议跨距传输心电图进行判读。

心电图的波形是基于心脏电流的变化（以毫伏测定）。标准心电图校准为 10mm/mV。因此，纵轴上 0.1mV 等于 1mm。为方便起见，在本文件中，心电图变化在校准后以 mm 表示。

在临床背景下，以下情况 ST 段抬高（在 J 点测量）提示进行性冠状动脉急性闭塞：至少 2 个相邻导联 ST 段抬高；在没有左室肥厚或左束支传导阻滞的情况下，$V_2 \sim V_3$ 导联 ST 段抬高在＜ 40 岁男性≥ 2.5mm、≥ 40 岁男性≥ 2.0mm、女性≥ 1.5mm，其他导联抬高≥ 1mm。下壁心肌梗死患者建议记录并观察右胸前导联（V_3R 和 V_4R）ST 段抬高情况，以识别是否伴发右心室心肌梗死。同样，$V_1 \sim V_3$ 导联 ST 段压低也提示心肌缺血，特别是当 T 波终末部分直立时（等同于 ST 段抬高），应当同时记录 $V_7 \sim V_9$ 导联心电图并确认是否伴有 ST 段抬高≥ 0.5mm，以便确定是否合并后壁心肌梗死。心电图出现病理性 Q 波不一定要改变再灌注决策。

有些病例的心电图诊断可能比较困难。尽管如此，也应当尽快予以处理和分诊。具体包括：

（1）**束支传导阻滞**　在左束支传导阻滞（LBBB）的情况下心电图诊断急性心肌梗死较为困难。但是 ST 段明显异常时通常可以作出诊断。有学者提出的诊断标准对诊断可能有帮助，不过该标准有点复杂，也不能保证确诊。出现同向性 ST 段抬高（即在正向 QRS 波群导联）可能是冠状动脉闭塞导致进行性心肌梗死的最佳指标之一。不论既往是否存在 LBBB，临床怀疑进行性心肌缺血合并 LBBB 的患者应当视为等同于 STEMI 并进行处理。需要指出，新发（或推测为新发）的 LBBB 本身并不预示心肌梗死。

心肌梗死合并右束支传导阻滞（RBBB）的患者预后不良。当患者存在胸痛和 RBBB 时诊断透壁性心肌缺血可能比较困难。因此，当患者出现持续性缺血症状并伴有 RBBB 时，应考虑采取 PPCI 策略（急诊冠状动脉造影并在有指征时行 PCI）。

（2）**心室起搏**　起搏器心律可能会妨碍对 ST 段改变的判读。这时可能需要紧急进行冠状动脉造影来确诊并启动治疗。对心室起搏没有依赖性的患者，在不延误有创检查的前提下，可以考虑进行起搏器程控，以便观察患者在自身心律状态下的心电图变化。

（3）**非诊断性心电图**　部分急性冠状动脉闭塞的患者可能早期心电图没有 ST 段抬高。有时是因为症状发作后极早期行的心电图检查，此时应当查找超急性期 T 波改变（可以进展为 ST 段抬高）。重复心电图检查或监测 ST 段动态变化非常重要。此外，有些冠状动脉急性闭塞和进行性心肌梗死的患者（如回旋支闭塞、静脉桥血管闭塞或左主干病变）可能不表现有 ST 段抬高，从而导致不能及时予以再灌注治疗，造成大面积梗死和更坏的结果。将 12 导联心电图扩展至加做 $V_7 \sim V_9$ 导联可能会识别出其中一些患者。即便是心电图缺乏有诊断意义的 ST 段抬高表现时，只要怀疑存在进行性心肌缺血就是 PPCI 的指征。表 4-2 列举了存在进行性心肌缺血症状的患者伴有不典型心电图表现时应当启动 PPCI 的情况。

表 4-2　有进行性心肌缺血症状患者应采取直接 PCI 策略的不典型心电图表现

束支传导阻滞
LBBB 时能够提高 STEMI 诊断准确性的标准： · QRS 主波向上的导联同向性 ST 段抬高≥1mm · $V_1 \sim V_3$ 导联同向性 ST 段下压≥1mm · QRS 主波向下的导联反向性 ST 段抬高≥5mm 存在 RBBB 时可能会影响 STEMI 的诊断
心室起搏心律
右室起搏的心电图表现为 LBBB，以上标准同样适用于起搏心律时心肌梗死的诊断，但是特异性较差
孤立后壁心肌梗死
孤立性 $V_1 \sim V_3$ 导联 ST 段下压≥0.5mm 和后壁导联 $V_7 \sim V_9$ ST 段抬高（≥0.5mm）
左主干闭塞或多支血管病变导致的缺血
≥8 个导联出现 ST 段压低≥1mm，同时伴有 aVR 和（或）V_1 导联 ST 段抬高提示左主干或左主干等同冠脉阻塞及严重的三支病变

注：LBBB：左束支传导阻滞；RBBB：右束支传导阻滞；STEMI：ST 段抬高型心肌梗死。

（4）孤立性后壁心肌梗死　下壁和基底部急性心肌梗死通常对应于回旋支病变，孤立性 $V_1 \sim V_3$ 导联 ST 段压低≥0.5mm 是最常见的表现。这种情况应当按照 STEMI 予以处理。建议加做后胸壁导联（$V_7 \sim V_9$ 导联抬高≥0.5mm，40 岁男性≥1mm）以便发现下壁和基底部 STEMI。

（5）左主干闭塞　在≥6 个体表心电图导联出现 ST 段压低≥1mm（下侧壁 ST 段压低），同时伴有 aVR 和（或）V_1 导联 ST 段抬高，提示多支血管缺血或左主干阻塞（尤其是存在血流动力学的改变时）。

有必要在急性期常规取血进行血清标志物检测，但不能因此而延迟再灌注策略或治疗。

如果对急性演变期心肌梗死的诊断有疑问，急诊影像学检查有助于为这些患者的及时再灌注治疗提供支持。超声心动图用于初步诊断的建议见第六章第 6 节。没有条件进行超声心动图检查或超声心电图检查结果不确定时，应行 PPCI（患者在非 PCI 中心接受初始治疗时，应立即转运至 PCI 中心）。

对于急诊 STEMI 患者，常规进行计算机体层扫描（CT）没有价值。CT 仅限于怀疑急性主动脉夹层或肺栓塞时有选择使用。STEMI 诊断几乎肯定时，不建议进行 CT 检查。

一些非急性心肌梗死病症可以出现与 STEMI 类似的症状和心电图改变，这时建议行急诊冠状动脉造影进行鉴别（详见第九章）。

第 2 节　减轻疼痛、呼吸困难和焦虑

缓解疼痛非常重要。这不仅是出于舒适和安慰目的，还在于疼痛与交感神经兴奋有关，后者可造成血管收缩和心脏负担加重。静脉注射阿片类药物（如吗啡）是目前最常用的镇痛方法（表 4-3）。不过，吗啡可引起口服抗血小板药物（氯吡格雷、替格瑞洛和普拉格雷）吸收减缓、起效延迟和药效减弱，对于某些敏感患者可能会造成其早期治疗的失败。

表 4-3　缓解低氧血症和症状

建议	建议类别	证据水平
低氧血症		
氧疗只用于低氧血症的患者（$SaO_2 < 90\%$ 或者 $PaO_2 < 60mmHg$）	I	C
$SaO_2 \geq 90\%$ 的患者不建议常规氧疗	Ⅲ	B
症状		
应该考虑静脉使用适当剂量的阿片类药物缓解疼痛	Ⅱa	C
应该考虑使用弱镇静剂（通常是苯二氮䓬类）治疗明显焦虑的患者	Ⅱa	C

注：SaO_2：动脉血氧饱和度；PaO_2：动脉氧分压。

动脉血氧饱和度（SaO_2）< 90% 是低氧血症患者进行氧疗的指征。有证据显示组织氧过多可能加重心肌损伤，对没有并发症的心肌梗死患者不利。因此，SaO_2 ≥ 90% 时不建议常规氧疗。

焦虑是对疼痛及发生心肌梗死时周围环境的自然反应。因此，对患者和与其密切相关的人进行安抚非常重要。

焦虑患者可以考虑使用弱镇静剂（常用苯二氮䓬类）。

第3节　心脏骤停

许多死亡发生在 STEMI 发病极早期，原因为心室颤动（室颤）。这种心律失常多发生于早期，因而大多数室颤发生在院外。因此，对疑诊心肌梗死患者进行救治的医疗和医疗辅助人员必须携带除颤设备并有能力进行心脏生命支持。FMC 时应立即对所有疑诊心肌梗死的患者进行心电监测。

应提高公众意识，引导公众在出现提示心肌梗死的胸痛症状时呼叫并等待 EMS 将其转运至医院救治。

心脏骤停后的患者如有心电图 ST 段抬高，应选择 PPCI。

由于心脏骤停患者中冠状动脉闭塞的发生率高，并且心脏骤停后心电图判读难度较大，建议对高度怀疑进行性心肌梗死（如心脏骤停前出现胸痛、既往确诊冠心病史，以及有异常或难以确诊的心电图表现）或无反应的幸存者进行紧急冠状动脉造影（2小时内）。对于没有 ST 段抬高的患者，在急诊室或心脏重症监护病房进行快速评估以排除非冠状动脉病因（脑血管事件、呼吸衰竭、非心源性休克、肺栓塞和中毒），并可以进行急诊超声心动图检查（表4-4）。决定采取紧急冠状动脉造影和必要时 PCI 策略时，需要顾及与神经系统不良后果相关的因素。提示神经系统功能恢复希望渺茫的院前不利因素包括：非目击的心脏骤停、院前急救团队到达不及时且没有外行进行基本生命支持（超过 10min）、初始存在不可电击复律心律，以及超过 20min

表 4-4　心脏骤停处理建议

建议	建议类别	证据水平
心脏骤停复苏成功的患者心电图提示 STEMI 时实施直接 PCI	I	B
心脏骤停心肺复苏后仍无反应的患者建议早期实施目标化体温管理[a]	I	B
建议医疗系统采取措施，促进通过一个专业的 EMS 系统直接将所有疑诊心肌梗死患者运输至 24 小时 7 天不间断实施 PCI 再灌注的医院	I	C
建议所有医务人员和医疗辅助人员救治疑诊心肌梗死患者时配置除颤设备并具备基础心脏生命支持技能	I	C
对于心脏骤停复苏后高度怀疑进行性心肌缺血的患者，尽管没有诊断意义的 ST 段抬高，也应该考虑实施紧急冠状动脉造影（必要时 PCI）	II a	C
不建议在院前对自主循环恢复后的患者立即快速输注大量低温液体降低体温	III	B

注：STEMI：ST 段抬高型心肌梗死；EMS：急救医疗系统；PCI：经皮冠状动脉介入治疗。

[a] 目标化体温管理是指采用主动的办法（如使用冷却导管、冷却毯、在患者身体周围放置冰块等法），使患者体温达到 32℃～36℃ 并维持一段时间（通常 ≥ 24 小时）。

的高级生命支持但仍未恢复自主循环。此时强烈提示不采取冠状动脉有创诊疗策略。

　　送至重症监护病房时仍处于昏迷状态的院外心脏骤停患者死亡风险高，幸存者中神经功能缺损常见。心脏骤停（或推测为心脏原因）复苏后仍处于昏迷状态是目标化体温处理的指征，即低温治疗。将体温持续控制在 32℃～36℃ 范围至少 24 小时。然而，低体温条件下口服抗血小板药物（氯吡格雷、替格瑞洛和普拉格雷）的吸收减慢、起效延迟，并且药效减弱。此外，低体温时氯吡格雷肝脏内代谢转化减慢。低温治疗不应推迟 PPCI，可以在导管室中同步进行。低体温患者需密切关注其抗凝问题。

　　预防并提高院前心脏骤停的救治水平是降低冠状动脉疾病相关死亡率的关键。详细讨论叙述请参考近期欧洲复苏委员会制定的复苏指南。

第4节　院前治疗后勤保障

1. 延迟

治疗延迟是 STEMI 患者医疗质量中最容易评估的指标。每个 STEMI 救治系统都应记录治疗延迟信息并定期检查，以确保这些简便的医疗质量指标达标并得以保持（见第十章）。如果不能实现设定的时间目标，应采取干预措施改进。缺血时间的构成、初步诊治的延迟、血运重建策略的选择见图4-1。

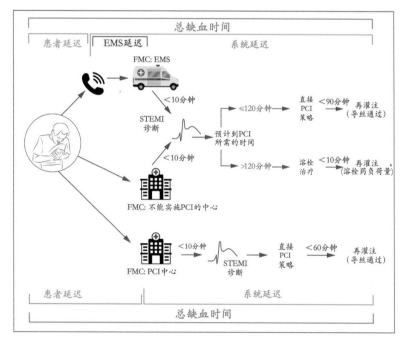

图4-1　患者就诊模式、缺血时间的组成和再灌注治疗策略的流程图

注：EMS：急救医疗系统；FMC：首次医疗接触；PCI：经皮冠状动脉介入治疗；STEMI：ST 段抬高型心肌梗死。

患者就诊的推荐模式为呼叫 EMS（呼叫国家急救电话号码：112 或类似号码）。如果在院外（如EMS）或非 PCI 中心诊断 STEMI，需要依据预计的从 STEMI 诊断到 PCI 导丝通过病变之间的时间来选择再灌注策略。对于呼叫 EMS 的患者，系统延迟计时开始于拨打电话的时间点，尽管 FMC 发生在 EMS 到达现场时（见表4-5）。

ᵃ 溶栓患者推注溶栓剂负荷量后应立即转运至 PCI 中心。

为了减少患者就诊延迟，建议提高公众对急性心肌梗死常见症状的识别能力和呼叫急救服务的意识。代表医疗质量的系统延迟因素和建议的医疗质量评估指标见第十章。

院内与急救系统人员救治 STEMI 患者的目标是缩短 FMC 到 STEMI 诊断的时间（≤10min）。STEMI 诊断是指判读心电图为 ST 段抬高（或等同情况）的那个时间点，也是治疗的起点。

与患者自身因素延迟比较，系统延迟更容易通过组织措施来缩短，它是结果的一个预测因素。

当院前 EMS 作出 STEMI 诊断后立即启动导管室不仅能减少治疗延迟，还能降低患者死亡率。由 EMS 做出 STEMI 诊断并准备运送患者进行 PPCI 时，可以绕过急诊室将患者直接送到导管室。绕过急诊室可使 FMC 到导丝通过病变时间缩短 20min。门进门出时间（door-in to door-out time）是一个新质量评价指标，是指患者转运 PCI 过程中患者到达非 PCI 中心医院至办理出院的时间。为了快速完成再灌注治疗，建议控制门进门出时间≤30min。

2. 医疗急救系统

EMS 使用便于宣传和记忆的医疗调度号码对于迅速启动急救至关重要（112 是大多数欧洲医疗急救电话）。应当避免绕过 EMS 对 STEMI 患者进行转运。救护车在 STEMI 患者的早期诊治中占有重要地位。它不仅是一种运送方式，也是一个强化早期诊断、分诊和治疗的系统。

所有救护车均需配备心电图机和除颤仪，并且至少有 1 人能够进行高级生命支持。院前救治的质量取决于救护人员的受训程度。救护车成员应当能识别急性心肌梗死症状，必要时进行氧疗、镇痛和提供基本生命支持。救护人员应当能够记录心电图，能够判读心电图或向冠心病监护病房、心脏重症监护病房或其他部门有经验的医师传输心电图，以便做出 STEMI 诊断。医疗辅助人员经过训练能够安全有效地为患者输注溶栓药物。对于发病早期患者，当预计从 STEMI 诊断到 PCI 再灌注时间超过 120min 时应予以院前溶栓治疗。因此，即便是在当前 PPCI 时代，也应当培训医疗辅助人员掌握溶栓技能。

3. STEMI 救治网络的建立

STEMI 的优化治疗应当依靠由不同技术水平的医院组成的辐射状网络（轮轴和轮辐）和优先、高效的救护车服务。这些网络的目标是提供最佳医疗服务的同时将延迟最小化，从而改善临床结局。心脏专科医师应当积极与所有相关人员尤其是急诊科协作，来建立这种网络。该网络的主要特征有：

- 明确的地域职责。
- 救护车或直升机中受过训练的医师、护士或医疗辅助人员共享基于危险分层和转运的书面协议。
- 院前将 STEMI 分诊至适宜医疗机构，绕开非 PCI 医院或不具备 24 小时 7 天不间断 PPCI 能力的医院。
- 到达适宜医院时，立即将患者送至导管室，绕开急诊室。
- 送至非 PCI 医院等待转运 PPCI 或补救性 PCI 的患者，必须在配备有监护设备和医疗人员的区域予以看护。
- 若救护车将患者送至没有 PCI 条件的医院并且工作人员没有做出 STEMI 诊断时，救护车应当等待患者的诊断。一旦 STEMI 诊断确立，应继续运送患者至有 PCI 能力的医院。

为了使成员的经验最大化，PPCI 中心应当 24 小时 7 天不间断为所有 STEMI 患者提供系统性 PCI 操作。也可以采用其他模式（尽管不太理想），包括同一区域内 PPCI 中心隔日或隔周轮换值班或设立多个 PPCI 中心。不具备 24 小时 7 天不间断 PPCI 能力医院，允许其对因其他原因住院期间发生 STEMI 的患者实施 PPCI。然而，要限制这些医院开展仅限于白天的 PPCI 或者开展耗时数小时的 PPCI，因为这样做会使 EMS 人员感到迷惑，对从诊断到再灌注治疗的时间和真正提供 24 小时 7 天不间断服务的 PCI 中心的介入治疗质量产生影响。因此，EMS 应将 STEMI 患者运送至已经建立 24 小时 7 天不间断心脏病介入治疗项目的医院，必要时可以绕开没有 PCI 能力的医院（如果转运时间在 PPCI 建议的时间窗范围之内）（图 4-2）。

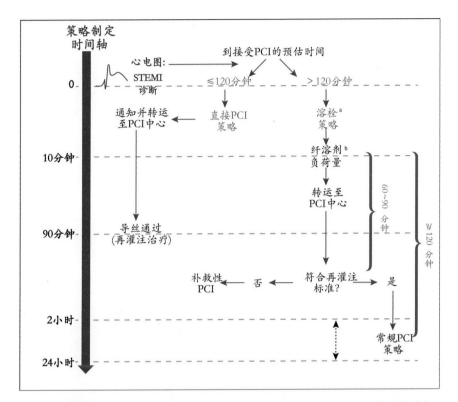

图 4-2　通过 EMS 就诊或就诊于非 PCI 中心的患者再灌注治疗策略的选择

注：PCI：经皮冠状动脉介入治疗；STEMI：ST 段抬高型心肌梗死。

STEMI 诊断位于策略制定时间轴的 0 时。通过 EMS 就诊（院外）或就诊于非 PCI 中心的患者，再灌注治疗策略依据预估的从 STEMI 诊断到 PCI 再灌注导丝通过病变之间的时间来决定。从 STEMI 诊断开始的目标时间代表进行相应干预的最大时间。

[a] 如果有溶栓禁忌，不论到 PCI 的所需时间长短，实施直接 PCI 策略。

[b] 10min 是从 STEMI 诊断到给予溶栓剂负荷量的最长目标时间延迟；但是在 STEMI 诊断后应尽快给予溶栓治疗（在排除禁忌证后）。

　　由于地域限制，预计转运至 PPCI 中心的所需时间超过建议的时间延迟范围时，应当建立在 STEMI 诊断地点立即进行溶栓、然后迅速转运至 PCI 中心的体制（图 4-1）。这样的网络系统可以提高再灌注患者中最短治疗延迟者的比例。应定期对医疗质量、时间延迟、患者结局进行分析比较，以便于改进。

4. 全科医师

在某些国家，全科医师在急性心肌梗死患者的早期救治中起着作用，通常也是患者最早联系的医师。如果全科医师能够迅速做出反应那将会是非常有效的，因为全科医师通常了解患者情况，并能记录和判读心电图。他（她）们作出 STEMI 诊断后的首要任务应当是联系 EMS。此外，全科医师可以给患者使用阿片类和抗血栓药物（包括有溶栓指征时进行溶栓治疗），必要时还可以实施电除颤。然而，大多数情况下先求助于全科医师而不是直接拨打 EMS 会增加院前延迟。因此，通常应当教育公众在出现可疑心肌梗死症状时首先呼叫 EMS，而不是呼叫初级保健医师。

表 4-5 院前急救的调度

建议	建议类别	证据水平
应依靠旨在快速有效地提供再灌注治疗的区域网络对 STEMI 患者进行院前救治，为尽可能多的患者实施直接 PCI	I	B
有直接 PCI 能力的医疗中心应提供 24 小时 7 天不间断服务，并且能够毫不延迟地实施直接 PCI	I	B
患者转运到具有 PCI 能力的中心时应该绕过急诊室和 CCU（或 ICCU），直接送达导管室	I	B
救护团队应具备识别 STEMI 的素质和设备（心电记录仪、必要时心电传输设备），有能力进行包括溶栓在内的初始治疗	I	C
建议所有参与 STEMI 患者救治的医院和 EMS 对延误时间进行记录和审核，并努力实现并保持医疗质量目标	I	C
建议 EMS 将 STEMI 患者运送到具有 PCI 能力的医疗中心，绕过非 PCI 中心	I	C
建议 EMS、急诊室和 CCU（或 ICCU）制定及并及时更新 STEMI 管理手册，最好能在区域救治网络内共享	I	C
送至非 PCI 医院等待转运直接 PCI 或补救性 PCI 的患者，必须安置在合适区域予以看护（如急诊室、CCU、ICCU 或者过渡监护病房）	I	C

注：CCU：冠心病监护病房；EMS：急救医疗系统；ICCU：重症心脏监护病房；PCI：经皮冠状动脉介入术；STEMI：ST 段抬高型心肌梗死。

⊕ | 评 注

本章讨论了 STEMI 的初步诊断、一般即刻处理、心脏骤停和院前治疗网络 4 个方面的问题。

在初步诊断中,指南强调了首次医疗接触时间(FMC)和如何快速诊断与鉴别诊断,其目的是为了让患者在最短时间内接受再灌注治疗,最大程度保护心肌,降低死亡率和心力衰竭发生率。然而,在美国和欧洲,FMC 几乎已经做到了极致,但是为经选择的 STEMI 急诊介入治疗死亡率仍然高达 7% 左右,心力衰竭发生率更高。要改变这种状况的另一项最重要的途径是进一步加强公共教育,最大程度缩短患者发病到呼叫医疗急救系统的时间。

ECG 诊断 STEMI 是再灌注策略的时间起点。患者应当接受 PPCI 策略。如果预计 STEMI 诊断到 PCI 再灌注绝对时间 > 120 分钟,则应立即开始溶栓治疗(即在诊断 STEMI 后 10min 内)。

尽早开始再灌注治疗的目的是为了挽救更多濒死心肌。新版指南提出的在首次医疗解除后 90min 内应当开通梗死相关血管。然而,实验研究显示,心肌持续缺血 > 30min,即开始发生不可逆坏死。因此,新版指南提出的时间概念只是一个最基本的要求,应当提出越快越好。

某些情况下患者可能在没有特征性 ST 段抬高,如束支阻滞、心室起搏、超急性 T 波、前壁导联孤立性 ST 段下移和(或)aVR 导联 ST 段抬高伴广泛前壁导联 ST 段压低,但是有冠状动脉闭塞和广泛心肌缺血。在有前述 ECG 变化和同时有与心肌缺血临床表现的患者,应采取 PPCI 策略。由于这些患者的 ECG 表现不典型,一般临床医师对这些患者缺乏认识,导致这些患者没有或延迟接受再灌注治疗,临床预后较差。因此,要认识有非典型 ECG 表现的拟诊心肌梗死患者,及早行冠状动脉造影进行鉴别诊断,适时实施再灌注治疗,降低这些患者的死亡率。

减轻患者的疼痛和焦虑可以降低患者的交感神经兴奋性,因而可能限制心肌梗死的面积。国外应用吗啡较多，国内应用较少。许多研究显示，吗啡可能抑制 P_2Y_{12} 受体抑制剂的吸收，应用时应当引起注意。指南认为 $SaO_2 < 90\%$ 是低氧血症患者进行氧疗的指征，但是有研究认为应当将氧疗指征放宽到 $SaO_2 < 93\%$。国内常常给 STEMI 患者长期吸氧，然而有证据显示组织氧过多可能加重心肌损伤，对没有并发症的心肌梗死患者不利，因此应当引起注意。

心脏骤停是导致 STEMI 患者死亡的重要原因，因此需要有一套完整的应对措施。新版指南强调，对于心脏骤停患者应当尽快行冠状动脉造影和（或）急诊 PCI，同时注意保护中枢神经系统功能。应当尽快送复苏后 ST 段抬高的患者做 PPCI。在复苏后心电图没有 ST 段抬高但是高度怀疑心肌缺血患者，应在快速评估排除冠心病后送患者 2 小时内接受急诊冠状动脉造影。对所有患者，在考虑紧急冠状动脉造影的同时，还应当注意与神经系统结果不良相关的因素。实际上，STEMI 心脏骤停患者救治成功率低，并且救治成功后存活患者的并发症多（包括神经系统），是 PPCI 面临的重要挑战。新版指南提出的尽快实施 PCI、对拟诊心肌梗死患者行急诊血管造影鉴别诊断和保护心脏骤停患者神经系统功能 3 个原则，对中国同行的临床实践有指导意义。

协调院外急救系统与医院之间的衔接是治疗 STEMI 患者的核心。无论是采取 PCI 策略还是院前溶栓，院外急救系统应当将患者转运到全天候大手术量的 PCI 中心。在选择再灌注策略后，院外急救系统应当即刻通知 PCI 中心。转送患者应当绕行急诊科，直接到 PCI 中心。STEMI 的救治是一个系统工程，需要方方面面的协作，要有一个切实可行的高效路径。中国胸痛中心的建立、推广与完善正是这种努力的体现。然而，鉴于各个地区发展不平衡，中国的出路在于做强基层网络，提高救治效率。由于我国各个医院的具体情况不同，因此不宜一味提倡绕行急诊科直接到 PCI 中心的做法，但是要理解新版指南提出这个建议的初衷是为了缩短救治延误时间。AHA 制订了一套全国性院前治疗后勤保障系统的方案，并且提出了具体的要求。美国许多州、市又根据本地的实际情况，制订出当地的方案，并且提出较 AHA 更严格的标准。为了保证院前治疗后勤保障系统的有效性，质量控制十分重要，美国的做法是定期召开有关各方参加的方案执行情况汇报会，找到目前存在的问题，修改现行的方案，进一步提高后勤保障系统的效能。AHA 和美国各地的做法非常值得中国借鉴。

第五章 ⊕ 再灌注治疗

第 1 节　再灌注策略的选择

再灌注治疗相关术语的定义见表 5-1。

表 5-1　再灌注治疗相关术语的定义

术语	定义
首次医疗接触	医师、医疗辅助人员、护士或者其他接受过训练的医疗急救系统人员对患者进行最初评估的时间点。这些人员能够获得和判读心电图，并进行初步干预（如除颤）。FMC 可以是在院前，也可能是在患者到达医院时（如急诊室）
STEMI 诊断	有缺血症状患者的心电图判读为 ST 段抬高或等同表现的时间点
直接 PCI	不事先溶栓，直接对梗死相关动脉使用球囊、支架或其他适宜器械进行急诊 PCI
直接 PCI 策略	急诊冠状动脉造影并在有指征时对梗死相关动脉实施 PCI
补救性 PCI	溶栓失败后尽早实施急诊 PCI
溶栓后常规早期 PCI 策略	溶栓成功后的 2 ~ 24 小时进行冠状动脉造影检查，必要时对梗死相关动脉实施 PCI
药物有创策略	溶栓治疗联合补救性 PCI（溶栓失败时）或常规早期 PCI 策略（溶栓成功时）

经验丰富的心脏团队可以迅速地实施 PPCI（即从 STEMI 诊断到恢复再灌注的时间 ≤ 120min，图 4-1 和图 4-2），因而对于发病 < 12 小时的 STEMI 患者是首选的

再灌注治疗策略（表5-2）。经验丰富的心脏团队不仅包括介入心脏病专家，还应包括专业技术人员。在手术量大的医疗中心，PPCI患者的死亡率更低。真实世界的数据证实，手术量大的医疗中心PPCI的实施速度更快、死亡率更低。随机临床试验也显示，再灌注延迟时间相同的情况下，手术量大且临床经验丰富的医疗中心实施PPCI的死亡、再梗死和卒中的发生率低于溶栓治疗。然而，在某些情况下如果不能立即实施PPCI时，可以立即开始溶栓治疗。目前还不清楚究竟PCI时间延迟多少会

表5-2　再灌注治疗的建议

建议	建议类别	证据水平
缺血症状持续时间≤12小时伴有ST段持续抬高的患者都应进行再灌注治疗	I	A
在指定治疗时间窗内直接PCI策略优于溶栓治疗	I	A
STEMI诊断后不能及时行PCI时，对症状发作12小时内并且没有禁忌证的患者实施溶栓治疗	I	A
有可疑进行性缺血症状提示心肌梗死但不伴有ST段抬高的患者，具备以下至少1项表现时建议实施直接PCI： ·血流动力学不稳定或心源性休克 ·药物治疗不能控制的再发或进行性胸痛 ·威胁生命的心律失常或者心脏骤停 ·心肌梗死相关的机械并发症 ·急性心力衰竭 ·再发ST段或者T波动态改变，尤其伴有间歇性ST段抬高	I	C
自行或使用硝酸甘油后症状完全缓解并且抬高的ST段完全恢复正常（未再发症状或ST段抬高）的患者应早期（24小时内）进行冠状动脉造影	I	C
发病超过12小时的患者，当存在进行性提示缺血的症状、血流动力学不稳定或威胁生命的心律失常时，应实施直接PCI	I	C
对发病后就诊较晚（12～48小时）的患者，应该考虑实施常规直接PCI策略	IIa	B
发病超过48小时没有症状的STEMI患者，不建议对其闭塞梗死相关动脉实施常规PCI	III	A

抵消其相比于溶栓的优势。由于缺乏专门针对这 2 种策略的临床试验，对事后分析的研究结果进行解释时应当持谨慎态度。不同研究中计算的可能降低 PCI 获益的 PCI 时间延迟结果不一致，例如，60min、110min 和 120min 不等。根据注册研究的估计，降低 PCI 获益的时间延迟界限在住院患者中为 114min，在没有 PCI 资质医院为 120min。不过，这些数据都已年代久远，溶栓治疗的患者并没有接受可以改善其预后的常规早期冠状动脉造影。近期的 STREAM 研究（STrategic Reperfusion Early After Myocardial infarction）将发病早期不能即刻实施 PCI 的 STEMI 患者随机分为即刻溶栓（随后常规进行早期冠状动脉造影）或转运 PPCI 两组进行了比较。该研究中与 PCI 相关的时间延迟中位数为 78min，两组的临床结果没有差异。由于缺乏同时期用以比较的证据，本指南编写委员会认为还不能设置 PCI 优于溶栓的时间界限。为简单起见，本指南选择采用从诊断 STEMI 到 PCI 再灌注即导丝通过梗死相关动脉的绝对时间限定在 120min 之内，而不是设定 PCI 时间延迟优于溶栓治疗的时间界限。考虑到从诊断 STEMI 到推注溶栓药物的时间上限为 10min，因而 120min 的绝对时间实际相当于 110～120min 的 PCI 相对于溶栓的时间延迟。这与过去临床试验和注册研究中 PCI 时间延迟限制范围一致。

如果选择溶栓治疗，从 STEMI 诊断到推注溶栓药物不应超过 10min。这一时间是基于 STREAM 研究中从随机到推注溶栓药物的中位数时间（9min）得出的。在之前 ESC 的 STEMI 指南中，这一时间的目标是 30min，但这是从 FMC（而不是从诊断 STEMI）开始计算的。FMC 后应当在 10min 内诊断 STEMI（表 5-3）。

图 4-2 总结了院前或首诊于无 PCI 条件医院的患者的目标时间。

为了缩短再灌注治疗的时间，在可能的情况下（图 4-1 和图 4-2）应当进行院前溶栓。溶栓后应尽快将患者转运至有 PCI 条件的医院。补救 PCI 是指溶栓失败（即溶栓后 60～90min 的 ST 段回落率 < 50%）或者因血流动力学或电活动不稳定、缺血加重或持续性胸痛而进行的 PCI，而常规的早期 PCI 策略是指溶栓成功后进行的 PCI（最好是溶栓后 2～24 小时）。

当患者的临床表现高度怀疑急性心肌梗死，但是心电图表现为不能解释的 ST 段改变时，如束支阻滞或心室起搏，应当采取 PPCI 策略。

表 5-3　重要目标时间总结

时间	时间目标
从首次医疗接触至心电图检查和诊断的最长间隔 [a]	≤ 10min
直接 PCI 策略优于溶栓治疗的最大预计时间延迟（从 STEMI 确诊到直接 PCI 导丝通过病变的时间间隔），如果超过该目标则考虑溶栓治疗	≤ 120min
就诊于能够行直接 PCI 医院的患者从 STEMI 诊断到导丝通过病变的最大时长	≤ 60min
转运患者从 STEMI 诊断到导丝通过病变的最大时间间隔长	≤ 90min
不能达成直接 PCI 时间目标的患者，从 STEMI 诊断到溶栓药负荷量推注或开始溶栓药输注的最大时间间隔	≤ 10min
从溶栓开始到疗效评估（成功还是失败）的时间延迟	60 ～ 90min
从溶栓开始到冠状动脉造影（如果溶栓成功）的时间延迟	2 ～ 24h

注：[a] 心电图需要立即判读。

　　通常认为，发病＞ 12 小时的患者出现以下情况时也应当进行 PPCI：①心电图提示持续性缺血；②持续或反复胸痛伴心电图的动态变化；③持续或反复胸痛伴心力衰竭、休克或恶性心律失常。然而，对于没有临床和（或）心电图证据提示持续性缺血的患者，PCI 是否获益尚不明确。一项小规模的（347 例）随机研究显示，对于发病 12 ～ 48 小时且无症状的患者，与单纯保守治疗相比，PPCI 可以挽救更多的心肌并提高患者的 4 年生存率。然而，OAT（Occluded Artery Trial）研究是一项大规模（2166 例）临床研究，结果显示，对于心肌梗死后 3 ～ 28 天并且梗死相关动脉持续闭塞的稳定患者，常规进行 PCI 与药物治疗相比并没有额外的临床获益。一项荟萃研究显示，晚期开通闭塞梗死相关动脉进行再灌注没有获益。因此，对发病＞ 48 小时无症状的患者不建议常规进行 PCI 开通梗死相关动脉。这些患者的治疗策略应当与所有慢性完全闭塞的患者一样，即仅当闭塞动脉供血区域存在存活心肌或出现缺血症状时，才应当考虑血运重建治疗。

第 2 节　直接经皮冠状动脉介入治疗和辅助治疗

1. 经皮冠状动脉介入治疗的术中事项

（1）穿刺途径

近年来，已有数项研究证据强烈支持桡动脉穿刺经验丰富的术者将其作为 ACS 患者 PPCI 时的首选途径。MATRIX 研究（Minimizing Adverse Haemorrhagic Events by TRansradial Access Site and Systemic Implementation of angioX）将 8404 例 ACS 患者（STEMI 患者占 48%）随机分为经桡动脉或经股动脉途径两组。结果显示，桡动脉途径患者的穿刺部位出血、血管并发症及需要输血的发生率更低。重要的是，RIVAL 研究（Radial Versus Femoral Access for Coronary Intervention）和 RIFLE-STEACS 研究（Radial Versus Femoral Randomized Investigation in ST-Elevation Acute Coronary Syndrome）显示经桡动脉途径患者的死亡率更低。MATRIX 研究没有观察到不同类型 ACS 之间的获益存在差异，因此相信其结论可以推广至 STEMI 患者。

1）支架在 PPCI 中的应用　冠状动脉支架技术可用于 PPCI。与单纯的球囊扩张血管成形术相比，金属裸支架可以降低再次心肌梗死和靶血管血运重建的发生率，但不降低死亡率。与金属裸支架相比，药物洗脱支架可以降低 PPCI 患者靶血管再次血运重建的发生率。

与第一代药物洗脱支架相比，新一代药物洗脱支架的安全性更好，有效性相似甚至更佳，尤其是支架内血栓和再次心肌梗死的发生率更低。近期 COMFORTABLE AMI 研究（Effect of biolimus-eluting stents with biodegradable polymer vs. bare-Metal stents on cardiovascular events among patients with AMI）和 EXAMINATION 研究（Everolimus-Eluting Stents Versus Bare-Metal Stents in ST Segment Elevation Myocardial Infarction）显示，急性心肌梗死患者中使用新一代药物洗脱支架效果优于金属裸支架，其获益主要来自于再次血运重建率的降低。最近公布的 EXAMINATION 研究 5 年随访结果显示，药物洗脱支架比金属裸支架的死亡率更低。NORSTENT 研究（Norwegian Coronary Stent）纳入了 9013 例接受 PCI 的患者（STEMI 占 26%），随机置入药物洗脱支架

或金属裸支架。在平均 5 年的随访中，两组之间主要终点发生率没有差异（全因死亡或非致命性自发性心肌梗死）。然而，药物洗脱支架组明确的支架内血栓（0.8% *vs*.1.2%；*P*=0.0498）和靶病变再次血运重建（16.5% *vs*.19.8%；*P* < 0.001）发生率均低于金属裸支架组。

已有研究调查 PPCI 时延迟置入支架是否可以作为减少微血管阻塞和保护微循环功能的一种方法。然而，近期两项小规模的研究显示，延迟置入支架后经心脏磁共振成像测得的微血管阻塞却是增加的。规模更大的 DANAMI 3-DEFER 研究（DANish Study of Optimal Acute Treatment of Patients with ST-segment Elevation Myocardial Infarction-Deferred versus conventional stent implantation in patients with ST-segment elevation myocardial infarction）纳入了 1215 例延迟置入支架（PPCI 48 小时后）的 STEMI 患者，主要临床终点（全因死亡、非致命性心肌梗死或因缺血对梗死相关动脉再次血运重建的联合发生率）并没有得到改善，常规延迟支架置入增加了靶血管再次血运重建率。基于以上的研究结果，不建议采用常规延迟支架置入策略。

2）血栓抽吸　多项小规模、单中心研究以及一项对 11 个小规模临床试验的荟萃分析显示，PPCI 时常规进行血栓抽吸能够获益。最近，两项大规模的（入组患者分别 > 10 000 例和 > 7000 例）随机对照研究显示，与常规 PCI 相比，常规的血栓抽吸并没有带来临床获益。由于增加了卒中发生率，TOTAL 研究（Trial of Routine Aspiration Thrombectomy with PCI versus PCI Alone in Patients with STEMI）（共入组 10 732 例患者）对血栓抽吸的安全性提出了警示。对高血栓负荷人群 [TIMI（Thrombolysis in Myocardial Infarction）血栓分级 ≥ 3 级] 的亚组分析显示，血栓抽吸可以减少心血管死亡 [170 例（2.5%）*vs.* 205 例（3.1%）；风险比 0.80，95%*CI*：0.65 ~ 0.98；*P*=0.03]，但是增加了卒中或短暂性脑缺血发作的发生率 [55 例（0.9%）*vs.* 34 例（0.5%）；比值比 1.56，95%*CI*：1.02 ~ 2.42，*P*=0.04]。

TASTE 和 TOTAL 研究中，1% ~ 5% 的患者由常规 PCI 组交叉至血栓抽吸组。基于这些数据和最近的荟萃分析结果，不建议常规血栓的抽吸；但是，当导丝通过或球囊开通血管后仍有大量血栓残留时，可以考虑血栓抽吸。

（2）多支病变的血运重建

STEMI患者中多支病变很常见（约占50%）。通常只对梗死相关动脉进行血运重建，是否需要同时对严重狭窄的非梗死相关动脉进行血运重建（预防性）尚存在争议。有研究显示，合并多支病变的患者PPCI术后的ST段回落率更低并且预后不良。美国国家心血管数据注册研究和纽约州立经皮冠状动脉介入治疗报告系统的数据显示，与只对梗死相关动脉进行血运重建相比，同时对非梗死相关动脉进行血运重建会增加多支病变患者的死亡率；但是，这些研究中，心源性休克患者都被排除在外。

与这个问题相关的随机临床试验的规模都很小（病例数为69～885例）。一项研究将214例合并多支病变的STEMI患者随机分为3组：只对梗死相关动脉进行血运重建组，同时对非梗死相关动脉进行血运重建组，分次对非梗死相关动脉进行血运重建组。结果显示，在平均2.5年的随访中，只对梗死相关动脉进行血运重建组的主要不良心血管事件（即死亡、再住院、因ACS再住院和再次冠状动脉血运重建）发生率最高。在这项研究之后，四项随机临床试验比较了只对梗死相关动脉进行血运重建和完全血运重建的差别，包括PRAMI研究（Preventive Angioplasty in Acute Myocardial Infarction）（465例，23个月随访）、CVLPRIT研究（Complete Versus Lesion-Only Primary PCI Trial）（296例，12个月随访）、DANAMI-3-PRIMULTI研究（Complete revascularization versus treatment of the culprit lesion only in patients with ST-segment elevation myocardial infarction and multivessel disease）（627例，27个月随访）和Compare-Acute研究（Comparison Between FFR Guided Revascularization Versus Conventional Strategy in Acute STEMI Patients With Multivessel disease）（885例，12个月随访）。在这些研究中，非梗死相关动脉的血运重建要么在PPCI术中进行（PRAMI和Compare-Acute研究），要么在住院期间分次进行（DANAMI-3-PRIMULTI研究），或者在出院前任何时间（即刻或分次）进行（CVLPRIT研究）。非梗死相关动脉实施PCI的指征为冠状动脉造影证实＞50%狭窄（PRAMI研究）、＞70%狭窄（CVLPRIT研究）或者由血流储备分数（fractional flow reserve，FFR）指导（DANAMI-3-PRIMULTI和Compare-Acute研究）。在所有四项研究中，完全血运重建都显著地降低了主要终点事件（联合临床终点）发生率，而总死亡率均无统计学差异。PRAMI研究、

DANAMI-3-PRIMULTI 研究和 Compare-Acute 研究显示，完全血运重建均显著地降低了再次血运重建率。仅在 PRAMI 研究中非梗死相关动脉血运重建组减少了非致命的心肌梗死。但是，三项荟萃分析显示，对非梗死相关动脉进行血运重建并不能降低死亡或心肌梗死的发生率。这些荟萃分析都没有包括 Compare-Acute 研究，其中一项荟萃分析没有包括 DANAMI-3-PRIMULTI 研究。基于这些研究的结果，出院前应当考虑对多支病变的患者非梗死相关动脉进行血运重建（表 5-4）。由于目前还没有充分证据证实何时为血运重建的最佳时机（即刻还是分次），因此，本指南对多支病变的患者进行即刻还是分次 PCI 没有优先建议。

表 5-4　直接 PCI 策略的技术操作问题

建议	建议类别	证据水平
梗死相关动脉策略		
建议对梗死相关动脉实施直接 PCI	I	A
对直接 PCI 后症状或体征再发、仍存在缺血症状或体征的患者，建议再次行冠状动脉造影，必要时行 PCI	I	C
梗死相关动脉技术		
直接 PCI 时应置入支架，优于球囊扩张血管成形术	I	A
建议直接 PCI 术应使用新一代药物涂层支架，优于使用金属裸支架	I	A
建议桡动脉途径操作熟练的术者实施直接 PCI 术时采用桡动脉途径，优于股动脉途径	I	A
不建议常规进行血栓抽吸	III	A
不建议常规行延期支架置入术	III	B
非梗死相关动脉策略		
出院前应当考虑对多支病变的患者非梗死相关动脉进行血运重建	IIa	A
心源性休克患者在直接 PCI 时应该考虑对非梗死相关动脉同期实施 PCI	IIa	C
患者有进行性心肌缺血且大面积心肌受累但不能对梗死相关动脉实施 PCI 时，应该考虑行 CABG 术	IIa	C

（3）主动脉内气囊反搏

CRISP AMI 研究（Counterpulsation to Reduce Infarct Size Pre-PCI-Acute Myocardial Infarction）显示常规的主动脉内气囊反搏（intra-aortic balloon pump，IABP）对无休克的前壁心肌梗死患者没有益处，反而增加出血。这与之前 IABP 在无心源性休克的高危 STEMI 患者中作用的研究结果一致。此外，最近的一项随机研究表明，IABP 并不能改善合并心源性休克的心肌梗死患者的临床结果。第八章讨论了心源性休克患者的血流动力学支持技术。

2. 围术期药物治疗

（1）抗血小板药物

接受 PPCI 的患者应当使用 DAPT（阿司匹林联合一种 P_2Y_{12} 受体抑制剂），再加上一种肠外抗凝药物。阿司匹林可以口服（包括嚼服）或者静脉推注，以确保完全抑制血栓烷 A_2 诱导的血小板聚集。普通阿司匹林（非肠溶制剂）的口服剂量最好是 $150 \sim 300mg$。静脉注射的最佳剂量缺乏相关临床资料。基于口服阿司匹林的生物利用度为 50%，因此，静脉注射的相应剂量为 $75 \sim 150mg$。药理学数据表明，低剂量的阿司匹林可以避免抑制环氧酶 -2 依赖的前列环素的生成。最近的一项随机研究显示，与 300mg 的阿司匹林口服相比，单次静脉推注 250mg 或 500mg 阿司匹林在 5min 时对血栓形成和血小板聚集的抑制速度更快、更彻底，并且不增加出血发生率。

STEMI 患者应当何时开始使用 P_2Y_{12} 受体抑制剂的证据尚不足。ATLANTIC 研究（Administration of Ticagrelor in the Cath Lab or in the Ambulance for New ST Elevation Myocardial Infarction to Open the Coronary Artery Trial）是唯一一项比较不同时间点给予 P_2Y_{12} 受体抑制剂对 STEMI 患者的安全性和有效性影响的随机研究。在这项研究中，患者被随机分组为转运至 PPCI 的医院之前给予替格瑞洛，或者在冠状动脉造影前即刻给予替格瑞洛。两种给药策略的平均间隔时间只有 31min，然而，这项研究未能达成预先设定的主要终点，即改善 ST 段回落率或 TIMI 血流。两种给药策略的严重和轻微出血发生率是相同的。尽管缺乏提前给予 P_2Y_{12} 受体抑制剂的临床证据，但是患者在被转运至 PPCI 的医院途中，早期给予 P_2Y_{12} 受体抑制剂在欧洲很常见，这与药代动力学的数据也是一致的。此外，观察性研究和一项小规模的随机试验证实早期给予高剂量的氯吡格雷优于在导管室内给药。总之，这些数据表明，提前给药（尤其对于再灌注延迟时间长的患者）可能更利于发挥其效果。然而，在 STEMI 诊断不明确的情况下，应当延迟给予 P_2Y_{12} 受体抑制剂的负荷剂量，直到检查明确冠状动脉解剖情况。

首选的 P_2Y_{12} 受体抑制剂是普拉格雷（60mg 的负荷剂量和 10mg，每天 1 次的维持剂量）或替格瑞洛（180mg 的负荷剂量和 90mg，每天 2 次的维持剂量）。这些药物的作用更快，效力更强，并且临床疗效优于氯吡格雷。由于缺乏临床净获益，既往有卒中或短暂性脑缺血发作的患者禁用普拉格雷；75 岁以上或体重较低（＜ 60kg）的患者通常不建议使用普拉格雷。如果这些患者需要使用普拉格雷，则应当减少剂量（5mg）。治疗初期替格瑞洛可能会引起短暂的呼吸困难，但是并不伴有肺的形态或功能性异常，并且很少因此而停药。既往出血性卒中、使用口服抗凝剂或者中重度肝病的患者禁用普拉格雷和替格瑞洛。

当没有普拉格雷或替格瑞洛，或者存在禁忌时，应给予氯吡格雷 600mg 口服。尚缺乏 PPCI 时比较氯吡格雷和安慰剂的大规模对照研究。CURRENT-OASIS 7 研究（Clopidogrel and aspirin Optimal Dose usage to reduce recurrent events-Seventh organization to assess strategies in ischaemic syndromes）显示，接受 PCI 的患者第一周使用 600mg 负荷剂量加 150mg 维持剂量优于 300mg 负荷剂量加 75mg 维持剂量。已证实高负荷剂量的氯吡格雷能够快速地抑制二磷酸腺苷受体。所有的 P_2Y_{12} 受体抑制剂都应当慎用于高危出血或严重贫血的患者。

坎格瑞洛是一种强效可逆的静脉 P_2Y_{12} 受体抑制剂，起效和失效都非常迅速。3 项随机对照研究在接受 PCI 的稳定型心绞痛或 ACS 患者中比较了坎格瑞洛和负荷剂量的氯吡格雷或安慰剂的效果。对这 3 项研究的荟萃分析显示，坎格瑞洛减少围术期的缺血性并发症，但是增加出血风险。这 3 项研究中的 ACS 患者均没有使用强效的 P_2Y_{12} 受体抑制剂（普拉格雷或替格瑞洛），STEMI 患者仅占 18%，因此其结论对于当前 STEMI 患者临床实践的适用性受限。然而，对于没有口服 P_2Y_{12} 受体抑制剂或口服药物不能吸收的患者，在 PCI 时可以考虑应用坎格瑞洛。

与常规在导管室内用药相比，院前常规使用糖蛋白 Ⅱ b/ Ⅲ a 受体抑制剂并不能获益，反而增加了出血风险。与比伐卢定相比，术中使用阿昔单抗＋普通肝素没有任何益处。糖蛋白Ⅱb/Ⅲa受体抑制剂可以作为冠状动脉造影证实大量血栓负荷、慢血流或无复流，以及其他血栓性并发症的补救性用药，但是这一策略缺乏随机试验的证据。总之，没有证据建议PPCI术中常规使用糖蛋白Ⅱb/Ⅲa受体抑制剂。冠状动脉内应用糖蛋白Ⅱb/Ⅲa受体抑制剂并不优于静脉应用。

（2）抗凝药物

可用于PPCI术中的抗凝药物包括普通肝素、依诺肝素和比伐卢定。OASIS 6研究（Organization for the Assessment of Strategies for Ischemic Syndromes 6）表明PPCI术中使用磺达肝癸钠有害，因此不建议使用。

尽管没有在PPCI中比较安慰剂和普通肝素的随机对照研究，大量的临床经验支持普通肝素的效果。建议PCI的标准剂量为初始推注70～100U/kg。没有足够证据支持使用活化凝血时间（ACT）来调整普通肝素的剂量或对其监测；如果测定ACT，不能因等待ACT结果而延迟开通梗死相关动脉。ATOLL研究（Acute myocardial infarction Treated with primary angioplasty and inTravenous enOxaparin or unfractionated heparin to Lower ischaemic and bleeding events at short- and Long-term follow-up）是一项纳入910例STEMI患者的随机非盲研究，比较了依诺肝素（0.5mg/kg静脉推注）与普通肝素对急性心肌梗死患者的缺血和出血事件的影响。依诺肝素并没有显著降低30天死亡、心肌梗死、手术失败或严重出血的主要联合终点发生率（相对风险减少17%，P=0.063），但是降低了次要联合终点（死亡、再次心肌梗死或ACS及紧急血运重建）的发生率。重要的是，没有证据表明与普通肝素相比依诺肝素会增加出血。ATOLL研究的一项方案分析中（占87%的研究人群），依诺肝素在减少主要终点、缺血终点、死亡率和严重出血方面优于普通肝素。对23项PCI临床试验进行的荟萃分析显示（30 966例患者，PPCI占33%），与普通肝素相比，依诺肝素显著降低患者的死亡率。这种获益对于PPCI尤其显著，可能与严重出血的减少有关。基于这些证据，STEMI时应当考虑使用依诺肝素。

5项随机对照研究在STEMI患者中专门比较了比伐卢定和普通肝素联合（或补救性使用）糖蛋白Ⅱb/Ⅲa受体抑制剂的效果。这些研究的荟萃分析显示，虽然比伐卢定减少了严重出血的风险，但是没有降低死亡率，反而增加了急性支架内血栓的风险。最近的 MATRIX 研究包括了 7213 例 ACS 患者（STEMI 占 56%），结果显示比伐卢定并没有降低主要终点（死亡、心肌梗死或卒中联合事件）发生率。比伐卢定的总心血管死亡率、出血发生率更低，但是明确的支架内血栓风险更高。最近发表的 STEMI 患者的亚组分析证实了 MATRIX 研究的结果与 ACS 的类型无关。MATRIX 研究表明，与仅在术中输注比伐卢定相比，PCI 术后延长比伐卢定的输注时间并没有改善临床结果。然而，一项事后分析表明，PCI 术后延长比伐卢定的输注时间（PCI 的维持剂量）的缺血和出血风险均为最低，这与比伐卢定药品说明书的用药方法是一致的。基于这些研究证据，STEMI 患者（尤其是高出血风险的患者）应当考虑使用比伐卢定。肝素诱导的血小板减少症患者建议使用比伐卢定。

PPCI 术后不建议常规抗凝治疗，除非有全剂量抗凝（如房颤、机械瓣膜或左心室血栓）或预防剂量抗凝（需要长期卧床的患者预防静脉血栓栓塞）的适应证。直接 PCI 患者围术期和术后抗栓治疗方案见表 5–5。

表 5–5　直接 PCI 患者围术期和术后抗栓治疗方案 [a]

建议	建议类别	证据水平
抗血小板治疗		
除非有禁忌证（如高危出血风险），建议在 PCI 术前或者至少在 PCI 时服用强效 P_2Y_{12} 抑制剂（普拉格雷或替格瑞洛）或者氯吡格雷（普拉格雷或替格瑞洛没药或对其有禁忌证时），并维持服用超过 12 个月	I	A
建议所有患者在无禁忌证时尽快口服或静脉推注（不能吞咽时）阿司匹林	I	B
发生无复流或者血栓并发症时，应该考虑使用糖蛋白 II b/ III a 抑制剂作为补救治疗措施	II a	C
未使用 P_2Y_{12} 受体抑制剂的患者可以考虑使用坎格瑞洛	II b	A
抗凝治疗		
在抗血小板治疗的基础上，建议所有患者直接 PCI 术中接受抗凝。	I	C

续表

建议	建议类别	证据水平
建议常规使用 UFH	I	C
发生肝素诱导的血小板减少症的患者，建议在直接 PCI 术中使用比伐卢定抗凝	I	C
应该考虑常规静脉使用依诺肝素	II a	A
应该考虑常规使用比伐卢定	II a	A
不建议磺达肝癸钠用于直接 PCI	III	B

注：ª 剂量方案见表 5–6。

表 5–6　直接 PCI 或未再灌注治疗患者的抗血小板和抗凝治疗药物剂量

直接 PCI 时抗血小板及肠外抗凝药物剂量	
抗血小板药	
阿司匹林	负荷量 150 ～ 300mg 口服，或 75 ～ 250mg 静脉推注（如果不能口服），维持量 75 ～ 100mg qd
氯吡格雷	负荷量 600mg 口服，维持量 75mg qd
普拉格雷	负荷量 60mg 口服，维持量 10mg qd。体重 ≤ 60kg 者建议维持量 5mg qd。普拉格雷禁忌用于既往脑卒中患者。不建议用于 ≥ 75 岁以上人群，若必须使用可以 5mg qd
替格瑞洛	负荷量 180mg 口服，维持量 90mg bid
阿昔单抗	0.25mg/kg 静脉推注，继之以 0.125μg/（kg·min）（最大剂量 10μg/min）输注 12 小时
依替巴肽	180μg/kg 静脉推注 2 次（间隔 10min），继之以 2.0μg/（kg·min）输注至 18 小时
替罗非班	25μg/kg 静脉输注（至少 3min），继之以 0.15μg/（kg·min）维持输注至 18 小时
肠外抗凝药	
UFH	若不使用糖蛋白 II b/ III a 抑制剂，则静脉推注 70 ～ 100IU/kg 负荷量 若使用糖蛋白 II b/ III a 抑制剂，则静脉推注 50 ～ 70IU/kg 负荷量
依诺肝素	0.5mg/kg 负荷量静脉推注

续表

比伐卢定	0.75mg/kg 负荷量静脉推注，继之以 1.75mg/（kg·h）静脉输注至术后 4 小时
未接受再灌注治疗患者抗血小板及肠外抗凝药物的剂量	
抗血小板药	
阿司匹林	负荷量 150～300mg 口服，维持量 75～100mg qd
氯吡格雷	负荷量 600mg 口服，维持量 75mg qd
肠外抗凝药	
UFH	与溶栓治疗时剂量相同（见表 5-8）
依诺肝素	与溶栓治疗时剂量相同（见表 5-8）
磺达肝癸钠	与溶栓治疗时剂量相同（见表 5-8）

注：qd：每天 1 次；bid：每天 2 次；IU：国际单位；PCI：经皮冠状动脉介入治疗；UFH：普通肝素。

3. 减少梗死面积和微血管阻塞的方法

梗死面积和微循环阻塞是 STEMI 存活者长期死亡率和心力衰竭的主要独立预测因子。微血管阻塞是指在成功地开通梗死相关动脉后仍存在心肌灌注不足，由多个因素导致。微血管阻塞的诊断标准为：PCI 术后即刻造影时 TIMI 血流＜3 级，或者当 TIMI 血流 3 级时心肌呈色分级为 0 或 1 分，或者术后 60～90min 时 ST 段回落率＜70%。其他诊断微血管阻塞的无创检查技术包括延迟钆增强心脏磁共振（目前识别和量化微血管阻塞的手段）、超声声学造影、单光子发射计算机断层成像（single-photon emission computed tomography，SPECT）和正电子发射断层成像（positron emission tomography，PET）。尽管临床前期和小规模临床试验证实多种治疗策略均有效，如冠状动脉缺血后适应、远隔缺血适应、早期静脉注射美托洛尔、糖蛋白Ⅱb/Ⅲa 受体抑制剂、针对线粒体完整性或一氧化氮通路的靶向药物、腺苷、血糖调节剂和低温治疗等。但是，目前仍然没有以减少缺血/再灌注损伤（心肌梗死的范围）为目标的治疗可以明确改善临床预后。减少缺血/再灌注损伤特别是微血管阻塞以进一步改善 STEMI 患者的远期心室功能，仍然是尚未解决的临床问题。

第 3 节　溶栓和药物有创策略

1. 溶栓的获益和适应证

在不能及时进行 PPCI 的情况下，溶栓是一种重要的再灌注治疗策略，每治疗 1000 例发病 6 小时内的患者可以减少 30 例早期死亡。包括老年人在内的高危人群在发病后 2 小时内溶栓绝对获益最大。对于发病 12 小时以内的患者，如果不能在诊断 STEMI 后 120min 内进行 PPCI，在没有溶栓禁忌时建议溶栓治疗（图 4-2）。患者就诊越晚（尤其是发病 3 小时后），越应当考虑转运行 PPCI（而不是溶栓）。因为随着发病时间的延长，溶栓的效果和临床获益会降低。存在溶栓禁忌证时，权衡溶栓的救命效果和潜在的致命不良反应十分重要。此时要考虑到其他可选的治疗措施，如延迟 PPCI。溶栓治疗建议见表 5-7。

表 5-7　溶栓治疗建议

建议	建议类别	证据水平
当溶栓作为再灌注治疗措施时，推荐在 STEMI 诊断后尽快实施，最好在院前进行	I	A
建议使用纤维蛋白特异性药物（替奈普酶，阿替普酶，瑞替普酶）	I	B
年龄 ≥ 75 岁人群使用替奈普酶时应该考虑剂量减半	II a	B
溶栓治疗时的抗血小板治疗		
建议口服或静脉使用阿司匹林	I	B
建议氯吡格雷联合阿司匹林	I	A
对于溶栓并随后进行了 PCI 的患者，建议 DAPT（阿司匹林联合一种 P_2Y_{12} 抑制剂[a]）至 1 年	I	C
溶栓治疗时的抗凝治疗		
建议溶栓患者同时接受抗凝治疗，直到血运重建（如果实施）或者到住院第 8 天。抗凝药有以下几种：	I	A
·依诺肝素静脉注射继之以皮下注射（优于 UFH）	I	A
·普通肝素：根据体重调整剂量，静脉推注负荷量继之以静脉输注	I	A

续表

·使用链激酶患者，抗凝药选择磺达肝癸钠静脉推注负荷量继之以 24 小时后皮下注射	Ⅱa	B
溶栓后转诊		
建议溶栓后立即将患者转运至有 PCI 能力的中心	I	A
溶栓后介入治疗		
对于心力衰竭或休克患者建议行急诊冠状动脉造影，有指征时行 PCI	I	A
当溶栓失败（60～90min 时 ST 段回落＜50%）、出现血流动力学或者心电活动不稳定，或心肌缺血加重时均建议行补救性 PCI	I	A
建议在溶栓成功后 2～24 小时进行冠状动脉造影，如有指征对梗死相关动脉实施 PCI	I	A
溶栓成功后再发心肌缺血或有证据提示血管再闭塞时，建议行急诊冠状动脉造影，必要时行 PCI	I	B

注：DAPT：双联抗血小板治疗；STEMI：ST 段抬高型心肌梗死；UFH：普通肝素。

[a] 溶栓后接受 PCI 术的患者可以选择氯吡格雷作为联合使用的 P_2Y_{12} 抑制剂；但接受 PCI 的患者在溶栓后 48 小时可以考虑换为普拉格雷或替格瑞洛。

表 5-8 列出了溶栓药物和联合抗栓药物的剂量。

表 5-8　溶栓和抗栓治疗时药物剂量

药物	首次治疗	禁忌证
溶栓药物剂量		
链激酶	30～60min 内静脉推注 150 万单位	使用过链激酶或阿替普酶
阿替普酶（tPA）	静脉推注 15mg 负荷量 30min 内以 0.75mg/kg 静脉输注（最多 50mg），随后 60min 内以 0.5mg/kg 静脉输注（最多 35mg）	
瑞替普酶（rPA）	2 次静脉推注各 10 个单位负荷量，间隔 30min	

续表

药物	首次治疗	禁忌证
替奈普酶（TNK-tPA）	单次静脉推注负荷量： 　体重＜60kg 时 30mg（6000IU） 　体重＜70kg 时 35mg（7000IU） 　体重＜80kg 时 40mg（8000IU） 　体重＜90kg 时 45mg（9000IU） 　体重＞90kg 时 50mg（10000IU） 75 岁以上患者剂量减半	
抗血小板药物剂量		
阿司匹林	初始剂量 150～300mg 口服，（不能口服时 75～250mg 静脉推注），维持量 75～100mg qd	
氯吡格雷	负荷量 300mg 口服，维持量 75mg qd 75 岁以上患者负荷量 75mg，维持量 75mg qd	
抗凝药物剂量		
依诺肝素	75 岁以下患者： 　30mg 负荷量静脉推注，15min 后每 12 小时皮下注射 1mg/kg，直到血运重建或至出院前最多 8 天。前 2 次皮下注射每次剂量不应超过 100mg 75 岁及以上患者： 　不进行静脉推注，首次皮下注射剂量为 0.75mg/kg，前 2 次皮下注射每次剂量最大为 75mg eGFR＜30ml/（min·1.73m^2）的患者，无须考虑年龄，均每天给药 1 次	
UFH	60IU/kg 负荷量静脉推注（最多 4000IU），继以 12IU/kg 静脉输注 24～48 小时（最多 1000IU/h）。目标 APTT 为 50～70s 或正常对照值的 1.5～2.0 倍，需要在第 3、6、12 及 24 小时监测	
磺达肝癸钠（仅用于使用链激酶患者）	2.5mg 负荷量静脉推注，继之以 2.5mg 每天 1 次皮下注射至出院或不超过 8 天	

注：APTT：活化的部分凝血活酶时间；eGFR：估计的肾小球滤过率；IU：国际单位；rPA：重组纤溶酶原激活剂；tPA：组织型纤溶酶原激活剂；UFH：普通肝素。

2. 院前溶栓

对 6 项随机试验的荟萃分析（6434 例）显示，与院内溶栓相比，院前溶栓的早期死亡率降低 17%，尤其是发病＜ 2 小时的患者。这些和更近的研究数据支持院前溶栓。STREAM 研究表明，对于发病＜ 3 小时的 STEMI 患者，如果不能在 FMC 后 1 小时内实施 PPCI，院前溶栓之后早期进行 PCI 与转运 PPCI 的临床结果相似。

如果训练有素的医疗人员或医疗辅助人员能够判读心电图，或者将心电图传输到医院让医师判读，则建议进行院前溶栓。目标是诊断 STEMI 后 10min 内开始溶栓。

3. 溶栓后的冠状动脉造影及经皮冠状动脉介入治疗

即药物有创治疗策略。开始溶栓后，建议尽快将患者转运到能够实施 PCI 的医院（图 4-2）。如果溶栓失败，或者有提示血管再闭塞或再梗死的证据如 ST 段再次抬高，则应立即行冠状动脉造影和补救性 PCI。没有证据表明在这种情况下再次溶栓获益，应当避免。即使溶栓可能成功（60 ～ 90min 内 ST 段回落率＞ 50%、出现典型的再灌注心律失常和胸痛完全缓解），在没有禁忌证时建议常规进行早期冠状动脉造影。一些随机试验和荟萃分析表明，与观察等待的策略（只有在患者出现自发的或诱发的严重缺血、左心室功能不全、门诊缺血试验阳性时才进行冠状动脉造影和血运重建）相比，溶栓后常规早期冠状动脉造影及随后必要时实施 PCI 可以减少再梗死和再发缺血。无论是哪个亚组的患者，溶栓后常规早期 PCI 均能够获益，并且不增加不良事件的风险（卒中或严重出血）。因此，建议将早期的冠状动脉造影和必要时 PCI 作为溶栓成功后的标准治疗（图 4-2）。

溶栓成功与 PCI 之间的最佳时间间隔是一个重要问题，临床试验的差异很大。从 CAPITAL AMI 研究（Combined Angioplasty and Pharmacological Intervention versus Thrombolytics ALone in Acute Myocardial Infarction）的平均 1.3 小时，到 GRACIA-1 研究（Grupo de Analisis de la Cardiopatla Isque´mica Aguda）和 STREAM 研究的 17 小时

不等。针对 6 项研究的汇总分析显示，溶栓后极早期冠状动脉造影（＜ 2 小时）不增加 30 天死亡或再梗死、住院期间严重出血的风险。从发病到冠状动脉造影的时间间隔更短（＜ 4 小时）可以减少 30 天和 1 年死亡或再梗死，以及 30 天的再发缺血。基于对此项研究的分析以及其他临床试验中溶栓到 PCI 的中位数间隔时间为 2 ～ 17 小时，建议在溶栓成功后 2 ～ 24 小时进行冠状动脉造影。

4. 溶栓药物的比较

应当首选纤维蛋白特异的溶栓药物。单次推注替奈普酶组织型纤溶酶原激活剂（TNK-tPA）（根据体重调整剂量）与 tPA 加速给药方案相比，降低 30 天死亡率的效果相似，而非脑出血和输血的发生率更低，更易于在院前使用。

5. 辅助抗血小板和抗凝治疗

早期研究表明溶栓药物（即链激酶）联合阿司匹林可以获益。首次给予阿司匹林应当采用嚼服方式或静脉推注，然后每天低剂量（75 ～ 100mg）维持。氯吡格雷联合阿司匹林可以降低溶栓患者的心血管事件和总死亡的风险，应当作为溶栓的辅助治疗。普拉格雷和替格瑞洛缺乏在溶栓患者中应用的证据。没有证据表明糖蛋白Ⅱ b/Ⅲ a 受体抑制剂能够改善溶栓患者的心肌灌注或临床结果，反而可能增加出血。

在完成血运重建之前最好都进行肠外抗凝，至少 48 小时或持续至出院前（最长不超过 8 天）。尽管增加了严重出血的风险，纳入 6095 例患者的 ASSENT 3 研究（ASsessment of the Safety and Efficacy of a New Thrombolytic 3）显示依诺肝素比普通肝素的净临床获益更大。在更大规模的涉及 20 506 例患者的 ExTRACT-TIMI 25 研究（Enoxaparin and Thrombolysis Reperfusion for Acute myocardial infarction Treatment-Thrombolysis In Myocardial Infarction 25）中对≥ 75 岁和肾功能受损的患者（估计肌酐清除率＜ 30ml/min）的患者使用了较低的伊诺肝素剂量。与根据体重调整剂量的普通肝素相比，依诺肝素降低了 30 天死亡和再梗死的风险，但是增加了非脑出血的发生率。依诺肝素的净临床获益（无死亡、非致命性梗死和颅内出血）更大。最后，大规模的 OASIS-6 研究显示磺达肝癸钠优于安慰剂或普通肝素，死亡和再梗死的发生率更低（尤其是链激酶溶栓的患者）。

一项链激酶溶栓的大规模试验显示，与普通肝素组相比，比伐卢定组 48 小时的再梗死率更低，但是轻微而非显著地增加了非脑出血的发生率。目前缺乏比伐卢定与纤维蛋白特异的溶栓药物联合应用的研究。因此，没有证据支持直接凝血酶抑制剂可以作为溶栓的辅助治疗。

抗栓"鸡尾酒"方案，即静脉推注替奈普酶（根据体重调整剂量）、口服阿司匹林和氯吡格雷、静脉推注依诺肝素之后皮下注射直至 PCI（血运重建），是药物有创策略中研究最为深入的部分。

6. 溶栓风险

虽然发生率低，溶栓显著增加卒中发生率（主要是脑出血）。溶栓后的第一天的风险尤其高。高龄、低体重、女性、既往脑血管病史、收缩压或舒张压升高等均为颅内出血的重要预测因子。最新的研究显示，颅内出血率为 0.09% ～ 1.00%。STREAM 研究显示，当替奈普酶的剂量减少 50% 后，≥ 75 岁患者的颅内出血发生率明显降低。多项研究显示，溶栓患者的非脑出血发生率为 4% ～ 13%。链激酶可能引起低血压，但严重的过敏反应罕见。由于链激酶抗体可能会影响其活性，并且会增加过敏的风险，因此，应当避免再次使用链激酶溶栓。

7. 溶栓禁忌证

耗时较短的成功复苏并不是溶栓的禁忌。溶栓对于难治性心脏骤停患者无效，并且增加出血风险，因此不建议使用。长时间或创伤性的成功心肺复苏出血风险增加，是溶栓的相对禁忌证。表 5-9 列出了溶栓的绝对禁忌证和相对禁忌证。

表 5-9 溶栓禁忌证

绝对禁忌证
既往颅内出血史或未知部位的脑卒中史
近 6 个月内发作过缺血性脑卒中
中枢神经系统损伤、神经系统肿瘤或动静脉畸形
近期出现过重大创伤、外科手术或头部损伤（近 2 个月内）
近 1 个月内有胃肠道出血
已知原因的出血性疾病（月经除外）
主动脉夹层
24 小时内接受过不可压迫的穿刺术（如肝脏活检、腰椎穿刺术）
相对禁忌证
近 6 个月内发生一过性脑缺血发作
口服抗凝药治疗中
妊娠或产后 1 周
难治性高血压［收缩压＞180mmHg 和（或）舒张压＞110mmHg］
晚期肝脏疾病
感染性心内膜炎
活动性消化性溃疡
长时间或有创性复苏

第 4 节 外科冠状动脉旁路移植术

梗死相关动脉通畅但冠状动脉解剖不适合 PCI、心肌梗死的范围大或者心源性休克的患者应当考虑急诊冠状动脉旁路移植术（coronary artery bypass graft surgery, CABG）。对于合并心肌梗死机械并发症且需要冠状动脉血运重建的患者，建议同时进行 CABG。在 STEMI 患者中，因 PCI 失败或冠状动脉闭塞但解剖不适合 PCI 而实施紧急 CABG 的情况并不多，因为在此种情况下外科血运重建是否获益并不明确。由于外科手术再灌注的时间延迟长，其挽救心肌改善预后的可能性降低而手术风险升高。

由于缺乏随机研究的证据，心肌梗死后病情稳定的患者择期 CABG 的最佳时机应当个体化。对加利福尼亚州出院数据的回顾性分析比较了心肌梗死后患者早期（＜3 天，4676 例）与延迟（≥3 天，4800 例）CABG 的效果。结果显示，早期 CABG 的患者死亡率高于延迟 CABG（未校正的死亡率为 5.6% *vs.* 3.8%；倾向性调整后的优势比为 1.40，95%*CI*：1.12 ～ 1.74；*P* ＜ 0.001），心肌梗死当天进行 CABG 患者的死亡率最高（8.2%）。NSTEMI 和 STEMI 患者之间没有任何区别，风险越高的患者越得到迅速治疗。血流动力学恶化或再发缺血事件高危的患者（即供应大面积心肌梗死血运的冠状动脉存在严重狭窄或反复缺血）应当尽快手术，而不必在停用 DAPT 后等待血小板功能完全恢复正常。对其余所有患者，DAPT 最好停用 3 ～ 7 天（替格瑞洛至少 3 天，氯吡格雷至少 5 天，普拉格雷至少 7 天），阿司匹林则建议继续使用。如果没有持续性出血，建议术后 6 ～ 24 小时后开始服用阿司匹林。

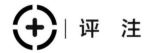

评 注

再灌注治疗策略是本指南的核心内容，我们重点评注。

STEMI 患者的再灌注治疗策略包括药物溶栓治疗、急诊 PCI 和急诊 CABG。然而，大规模研究显示，即使采用现代再灌注治疗，STEMI 患者 5 年病死率约为 10%，5 年心力衰竭发生率高达 70%。提示 STEMI 患者的治疗目标应当是包括尽快、充分和持续地开通梗死相关动脉（IRA）使其恢复前向血流在内的全程心肌保护治疗，降低患者的病死率和心力衰竭发生率。

选择何种再灌注策略时应当考虑就诊的医院和几个重要的因素。在可行 PCI 的医院，应当在入院后 90min 内完成急诊 PCI。在不能行 PCI 的医院，应当迅速评估：①症状发生的时间；② STEMI 相关并发症的风险；③药物溶栓发生出血的风险；④休克或严重心力衰竭；⑤转运到可行 PCI 医院的时间，即使医院间的转运时间非常短，立即溶栓的策略相对优于延迟进行急诊 PCI。超过 120min 进行 PCI 与立即溶栓比较，在生存率上没有优势。在没有禁忌证的情况下，预计 120min 以上才能进行 PCI 者，应当在 30min 内给予溶栓治疗。

目前，欧美指南已不再建议溶栓作为首选的再灌注治疗措施。但是，溶栓治疗快速、简便，在不具备 PCI 条件的医院或因各种原因使首次医疗接触时间（FMC）至 PCI 时间明显延迟时，对有适应证的 STEMI 患者，静脉内溶栓仍是较好的选择。院前溶栓效果优于入院后溶栓，有条件时可在救护车上开始溶栓治疗。对于发病 ≤ 3 小时的患者，溶栓治疗的即刻疗效与直接 PCI 相似，但是颅内出血风险增加。对于发病 3 ～ 12 小时的患者，溶栓治疗的效果劣于直接 PCI 并且出血性卒中风险增加。对于发病 > 12 小时的患者，溶栓治疗的获益不明确。对于发病 > 12 小时仍有症状而且缺血范围较大或血流动力学不稳定的 STEMI 患者，如果没有条件实施 PCI 时，专家共识支持进行溶栓治疗。

限于现实条件，目前溶栓治疗在我国仍然是一项重要的治疗措施，并且大部分地区多在医院内进行溶栓治疗。决定是否溶栓治疗时，应综合分析预期风险／效益比、发病至就诊时间、就诊时临床及血液动力学特征、合并症、出血风险、禁忌证和预期 PCI 延误时间。左束支传导阻滞、大面积梗死（前壁心肌梗死和下壁心肌梗死合并右心室梗死）患者溶栓获益较大。

溶栓治疗的主要缺点有：①溶栓患者致命性颅内出血发生率较高（0.5% ～ 1.5%）；②溶栓后 20% 的梗死相关动脉仍然闭塞，再通后还有 45% 梗死相关动脉的前向血流仅为 TIMI ≤ 2 级；③血管再通的中位数时间为 45min；④缺乏快速预测再灌注的指标；⑤ 15% ～ 30% 的患者再次发生心肌缺血。

优先采用特异性纤溶酶原激活剂。重组组织型纤溶酶原激活剂阿替普酶可选择性激活纤溶酶原，对全身纤溶活性影响较小，无抗原性，是目前最常用的溶栓剂。其他特异性纤溶酶原激活剂还有兰替普酶、瑞替普酶和替奈普酶等。非特异性纤溶酶原激活剂包括尿激酶和尿激酶原，可直接将循环血液中的纤溶酶原转变为有活性的纤溶酶，无抗原性和过敏反应。特异性纤溶酶原激活剂溶栓时需要抗凝支持以提高梗死相关动脉开通率并预防其再闭塞。

溶栓后只有冠状动脉恢复 TIMI 3 级血流的患者近期和远期预后得到改善，而 TIMI 2 级和 TIMI 0～1 级血流的患者预后相似。

溶栓后临床评估包括：

（1）ST 段回落　溶栓后抬高的 ST 段回落是心外膜动脉、微血管和组织水平心肌再灌注的一项标志。启动再灌注治疗后 60～90min ST 段回落 50% 以上提示再灌注。溶栓后 60～90min 内 ST 段完全或接近完全回落是梗死动脉再通的有用指标。相反，ST 段抬高部分改善或没有改善预测梗死动脉闭塞则缺乏准确性。研究显示，ST 段在 90min 回落 ≥ 70% 的患者中 TIMI 3 级血流者占 79%，ST 段部分回落和没有回落的患者 TIMI 3 级血流比例分别为 50% 和 44%。ST 段回落的程度和患者的近期、中期和远期预后相关。

（2）胸痛缓解情况　胸痛突然完全缓解伴有 ST 段最明显导联回落 > 70%，高度提示血流恢复正常。

（3）再灌注心律失常　如加速性室性自主心律、房室传导阻滞、束支阻滞突然改善或消失，或下壁心肌梗死患者出现一过性窦性心动过缓、窦房传导阻滞，伴或不伴低血压。最有价值的是加速性室性自主心律，但是其敏感性和特异性并不高。

（4）生化标志物　序列的心脏生化标志物监测可为溶栓后再灌注评估提供无创证据，如 cTn 峰值提前至发病 12 小时内，CK-MB 酶峰提前到 14 小时内。其中上升和下降都很迅速的 CK-MB 优于肌钙蛋白。然而，2013 年 ACC/AHA STEMI 未再提及生化标志物用于溶栓后再灌注的判断。这可能与指南要求溶栓后无论临床判断是否再通，均应早期（3～24 小时）进行旨在介入治疗的冠状动脉造影有关，在这种策略之下心脏生化标志物峰值对于判断溶栓再通已没有意义。

溶栓失败的冠状动脉造影定义为溶栓后 90min 时梗死相关血管持续性闭塞（TIMI 0～1 级）。TIMI 2 级或 TIMI 3 级为血管再通，TIMI 3 级为完全性再通。

溶栓治疗最主要的风险是出血，尤其是颅内出血（0.9%～1.0%），其中

1/2 ～ 2/3 是致命性的。65% ～ 77% 的颅内出血发生在溶栓治疗后 24 小时内。典型表现包括意识状态的改变、单部位或多部位的神经系统定位体征、昏迷、头痛、恶心、呕吐和抽搐发作，有时也表现为高血压急症。部分病例表现为迅速死亡。溶栓治疗后 24 小时内出现的任何神经系统症状都强烈提示颅内出血。可疑颅内出血时应立即停止溶栓、抗血小板和抗凝治疗。如果急诊 CT 和 MRI 确诊了颅内出血的类型和血肿定量，应该迅速采取降低颅内压的措施，同时考虑使用逆转溶栓、抗血小板和抗凝的药物。有颅内出血的 STEMI 患者应该请神经内科和（或）神经外科、血液科会诊。高龄、低体重、女性、既往脑血管疾病史、入院时血压升高、过度抗凝（国际标准化比值 INR ≥ 4，凝血酶原时间 ≥ 24s）和抗凝药物的选择（如阿替普酶比链激酶出血风险高）都是颅内出血的主要危险因素。

STEMI 患者 PCI 策略包括直接 PCI、补救 PCI、即刻 PCI、易化 PCI、延迟 PCI 和择期 PCI。急诊 PCI 的目的是尽快可靠地开通梗死相关动脉，重新建立有效的心肌灌注，达到挽救患者的生命并且改善其远期预后。其中，易化 PCI 由于概念的泛化，并且与直接 PCI 相比没有优势，目前不再主张使用。

规范 PPCI 技术对于提高手术质量十分重要。对于新版指南提出上述标准化要求，要有一个正确的认识。与中国患者比较，欧美患者身材和体重普遍较大，经桡动脉途径获益更多。经桡动脉途径在中国患者的应用比例更高，但是在 STEMI 患者经桡动脉路径并不妨碍使用大腔（例如 7F）指引导管。对于严重血流动力学或电活动不稳定的患者，还是应当优先选择经股动脉路径。新版指南建议的使用药物洗脱支架实施 PCI 是指的第 2 代药物洗脱支架，但是要注意，不同的第 2 代药物洗脱支架也存在差异。新版指南提出禁忌常规应用血栓抽吸，但我们对此持谨慎态度。欧洲的 STEMI 患者在发病后 2 ～ 3 小时就能接受再灌注治疗，而中国患者往往要在 6 小时后才接受再灌注治疗。研究显示，不同时间段的血栓构成不同。况且，血栓抽吸导管的功能不仅仅是抽吸血栓，并且还能为超选择冠状动脉内给药提供平台。实际上，在欧美专业学术会议病例演示时，鲜有不使用抽吸导管的情况。

根据体表心电图判断梗死相关动脉和病变部位，对于危险分层和预测术中可能出现的结果具有重要价值。例如左主干（LM）或左前降支（LAD）开口、近段急性闭塞的患者，即便术前没有发生左心衰竭和心源性休克，血管开通即刻或者术后也可能发生，往往需要采用药物和器械辅助来改善血流动力学状况。一般应先置入 IABP 再进行介入操作。右冠状动脉（RCA）尤其是近段急性闭塞患者血管开通后常出现缓慢性心律失常和低血压，无复流的概率也相对较高。

应当考虑急诊冠状动脉造影的情况包括：①适合直接 PCI 的患者；②适合血管重建治疗的严重心力衰竭或心源性休克患者；③有中、大面积心肌面临风险和有溶栓治疗失败证据的患者；④在血流动力学稳定并且有溶栓治疗成功证据的患者开始溶栓治疗后 3 ～ 24 小时。在开始没有接受直接 PCI 的不稳定患者（即严重心力衰竭或心源性休克和血流动力学受损的室性心律失常），应当实施旨在施行 PCI 的即刻冠状动脉造影策略，除非认为有创治疗对临床情况无益或不适合。

由于 PCI 术后不需绝对卧床，穿刺部位严重并发症发生率低，目前桡动脉途径已作为直接 PCI 的首选途径。然而，桡动脉途径优于股动脉途径的获益取决于术者桡动脉途径的技巧。此外，直接 PCI 术中随时可能出现血流动力学不稳定、心肺复苏等情况，腹股沟区应常规备皮、消毒铺巾，以备股静脉置管快速补液、输注血管活性药物、置入临时起搏电极或经股动脉行主动脉内气囊反搏术（IABP）。

6F 指引导管多数情况下可以满足直接 PCI 操作需要。桡动脉穿刺目前常用 6F 泰尔茂公司鞘管和强生公司鞘管。诊断性冠状动脉造影结果提示患者冠状动脉严重迂曲、钙化估计血栓抽吸导管或支架推送有困难，或分叉病变需要处理边支血管时，可以选择 7F 指引导管以增加支撑力或管腔直径。经 6F 鞘管置入普通 J 型导丝后将 6F 鞘管更换为 7F 鞘管。也可以改为股动脉途径置入 7F 鞘管。少数情况下桡动脉途径过度迂曲、发生血管痉挛导致指引导管难以推送或到位等情况，应迅速改为股动脉途径操作。

术前病情危重、血流动力学不稳定的患者，首选股动脉途径并常规使用 7F 鞘管。理由是：①股动脉穿刺相对简单迅速；②低血压状态动脉搏动不明显时可以盲法穿刺。盲法穿刺时，无论先穿刺到股动脉或股静脉均可，可以先置入导丝并以导丝为参照寻找股静脉或股动脉：先穿刺到股动脉时在导丝内侧 1cm 左右位置穿刺容易找到股静脉，先穿刺到股静脉时则在导丝外侧 1cm 左右位置穿刺容易找到股动脉。在股动脉和股静脉均成功置入导丝后，沿导丝切皮并先后将两个鞘管置入血管内；③

股动脉途径建议常规置入 7F 鞘管。危重患者通常需要股静脉鞘管补液、用药或置入临时起搏电极。股静脉内 7F 鞘管即便在置入临时起搏电极情况下也不影响补液速度；④股动脉相对粗大，常规使用 7F 指引导管可以避免遇到复杂病变时更换导管的操作，节省时间、保证手术成功率。必要时还可以使用 8F 鞘管。此外，左主干或左前降支开口病变需要对吻扩张时，也可以考虑首选股动脉途径。血流动力学不稳定、心功能 Killip 3 级、左主干或左前降支开口病变推测术中一旦发生无复流后果严重时，应先经左股动脉置入 IABP 再进行冠状动脉造影或介入操作。

原则上应该先进行罪犯病变对侧血管的冠状动脉造影。理由是：①目前首选经股动脉途径操作的患者多为病情危重，可以在完成对侧冠状动脉造影后直接采用指引导管进行罪犯病变侧冠状动脉造影。这样可以省去交换造影管的时间，进行 1 个或 2 个体位判断罪犯病变部位后可以马上进行介入操作。罪犯病变为左冠状动脉（LCA）时首选 7F JL4 指引导管，右冠状动脉则首选 7F JR4 指引导管。两者均为被动支撑导管，只要谨慎操作通常不必担心冠状动脉口损伤的问题。②经桡动脉途径操作时，也建议首先进行罪犯病变对侧血管的冠状动脉造影。有些情况下（如罪犯病变部位有造影剂滞留）仅推注 1 次造影剂就可能导致罪犯病变血流进一步恶化或完全闭塞。这时，如果事先完成了对侧冠状动脉造影，可以迅速更换指引导管开始介入操作。此外，对于病情较重的患者或经验较为丰富的术者，也可以在完成对侧冠状动脉造影后直接使用指引导管进行罪犯病变冠状动脉造影。

急诊冠状动脉造影时要注意以下问题：①考虑患者心功能受损问题，应尽量控制对比剂用量；在满足病变评估前提下，尽量控制造影体位数；②除了罪犯病变外，诊断性冠状动脉造影时留意其他冠状动脉病变情况也很重要，如钙化、迂曲等；③多支病变如有需择期处理的非罪犯病变，在血流动力学允许的情况下应获取必要的影像信息。

诊断性冠状动脉造影结果如为严重三支病变、左主干病变，即便患者血流动力学稳定也应先置入 IABP 后再进行 PCI 操作。少数单支病变患者冠状动脉造影即可造成血流动力学不稳定，这时也应先置入 IABP 后再进行 PCI 操作。

对于右冠状动脉一般采用左前斜和左前斜 + 头位摄像来显示右冠状动脉全程以

及与左冠状动脉供血范围的关系。血流动力学不稳定时只用左前斜 + 头位摄像。对于左冠状动脉 一般采用头位（或右前斜 + 头位）、右前斜 + 足位和左前斜 + 足位（蜘蛛位）三个体位摄像来显示左主干、左前降支 和左回旋支全程及其分支。血流动力学不稳定者首先采用右前斜 + 足位，如能满足病变判断随即进入介入操作。根据体表心电图判断为左回旋支闭塞的患者，诊断性造影体位选择基本同上。但有时需要增加足位摄像来显示左回旋支全程及其分支。对于左冠状动脉一般采用头位（或右前斜 + 头位）、右前斜 + 足位和左前斜 + 足位（蜘蛛位）三个体位摄像来显示左主干、左前降支和左回旋支全程及其分支。血流动力学不稳定者可采用头位（或右前斜 + 头位）、右前斜 + 足位（或蜘蛛位）两个体位。对于右冠状动脉一般采用左前斜和左前斜 + 头位摄像来显示右冠状动脉全程及其分支。开口至中段完全闭塞采用左前斜位置摄像即可。根据体表心电图判断为左主干病变的患者，投照体位基本同左前降支闭塞的体位。

直接 PCI 的优点有：①应用于不宜溶栓的患者，即扩大了治疗范围；②可以即刻了解冠状动脉解剖状况，同时评估左心室功能，因而可以进行早期危险分层；③迅速使梗死相关动脉再通，并且达到 TIMI 3 级血流；④心肌缺血复发、再梗死和再闭塞发生率低；⑤高危患者存活率较高；⑥心肌再灌注损伤和心脏破裂的发生率低；⑦致命性颅内出血风险降低；⑧缩短住院天数。

尽管 STEMI 直接 PCI 是一种抢救性的治疗手段，然而住院期间死亡率可以达 5%，因此，应当重视直接 PCI 术前、术中和术后的每一个环节，力求迅速、安全和有效。

经股动脉途径时，右冠状动脉首选 7FJR4 或 JR3.5，开口有病变时可自制 1～2 个侧孔。需要较强支撑时也可以使用 6F 或 7F SAL0.75、SAL1.0、XBRCA、AL0.75 或 AL1.0。左冠状动脉首选 7FJL4，左主干较短时也可使用 7F JL 短头（JL ST）指引导管。左前降支或左回旋支病变并且左主干正常时也可以使用 6F 或 7F EBU3.75 指引导管。当然，有些患者主动脉窦或主动脉较宽时可选择较大的指引导管，反之亦然。

经桡动脉途径时，右冠状动脉首选 6F JR3.5，开口有病变时可自制 1～2 个侧孔。需要较强支撑时也可以使用 6F SAL0.75、SAL1.0、XBRCA、AL0.75 或 AL1.0。左冠状动脉首选 6FEBU3.5，左主干较短时也可使用 6F JL3.5 或 JL 短头（JL ST）指引导管。

患者主动脉窦或主动脉较宽时可选择较大的指引导管，反之亦然。多数患者经桡动脉途径也可以置入 7F 鞘管。方法：先置入 6F 桡动脉鞘后置入造影导丝，保留造影导丝撤除 6F 桡动脉鞘然，再沿造影导丝置入 7F 下肢鞘。如有冠状动脉严重迂曲、器械通过困难，以及需要较多边支操作情况时可及时更换 7F 指引导管。

首选 BMW 指引导丝，也可以使用 Runthrough NS。直接 PCI 靶病变多为急性血栓形成导致冠状动脉闭塞，多数情况下 BMW 导丝能够通过病变。有时基础病变可能为严重狭窄、弥漫性狭窄、严重迂曲或钙化，BMW 或 Runthrough NS 不能通过病变。可以更换 Pilot 50 导丝或 Filder FC 导丝，通常能够顺利通过病变。指引导丝的塑形原则上制作小弯，向同一方向旋转（drilling）的方式通过病变。病变位于远端且近段血管角度较大或迂曲，指引导丝达到远端病变有困难时可做双弯，保证头端第一弯为小弯，容易通过罪犯病变。

指引导丝通过病变后，多数情况下冠状动脉血流仍不能恢复。因此，指引导丝操作过程中试注对比剂往往没有意义。这就意味着病变以远导丝的走行主要靠术者的经验判断。要求术者熟悉不同投照体位上各支冠状动脉的影像解剖，并且采用不同的投照体位来完成 PCI。实际操作过程中需要变换体位。例如，对于左前降支病变，首先需要采用右前斜 + 足位来显示近段解剖以便将指引导丝送至左前降支近段，然后变换到头位将指引导丝送至远端。对于左回旋支闭塞，采用右前斜 + 足位将指引导丝送至远端。对于右冠状动脉闭塞，先采用左前斜位将指引导丝送至中远段，然后采用左前斜 + 头位继续送至左心室后支或后降支。少数患者需要在球囊导管或微导管支撑下将指引导丝送至远端。

对于诊断梗死相关动脉完全闭塞或者非完全闭塞但血栓负荷明显的患者，笔者主张直接 PCI 时使用血栓抽吸导管。其理由是：①虽然目前对于直接 PCI 中使用抽吸导管是否有远期获益还存在争议，但是血栓抽吸改善术后即刻心肌灌注、减少远端栓塞或无复流的作用是肯定的；②多数情况下抽吸导管可以通过闭塞病变并成功开通闭塞病变而不需要预扩张。抽吸后进行造影多数情况下足以显示基础病变，能够满足对拟支架直径和长度的判断。③血栓负荷较重时，少数病例仅采用预扩张往往不能开通闭塞病变，从而导致因基础病变不可显示而不能置入支架。只有在充分进行血栓抽吸后才能清楚显示罪犯病变。

笔者不主张直接PCI时进行常规预扩张。预扩张应仅限于抽吸导管不能通过病变，或者罪犯病变为非完全闭塞病变但支架不能通过病变时使用。预扩张球囊的选择应为小于参考血管直径，不主张过高压力预扩张以避免增加无复流或远端栓塞的发生率（一般6～10atm即可）。

原则上直接PCI应置入支架而不是球囊扩张成形术，置入支架能够降低急性闭塞、再发梗死和再次血运重建治疗率。梗死相关动脉直径较小、病变解剖条件置入支架非常困难时，可以仅仅进行血栓抽吸或球囊扩张。置入支架应保证完全覆盖罪犯病变。STEMI时由于冠状动脉闭塞导致远端灌注压低，往往血管有收缩，因此，无论冠状动脉造影还是IVUS对血管直径的判断都有困难。可以参照病变近端直径选择支架。有明显冠状动脉痉挛发生或血压情况允许时，在血栓抽吸或球囊扩张后应向冠状动脉内推注硝酸甘油50～200μg或尼可地尔2～5mg或钙拮抗药消除冠状动脉痉挛因素，帮助评估罪犯病变的直径和长度，选择适合型号的支架。

STEMI罪犯病变无复流的发生率较高，原则上支架置入应避免不必要的预扩张或后扩张。支架高压释放（≥12atm），压力也不宜过高，一般12～14atm即可。如果支架直径合适且膨胀良好时，可不必进行后扩张。然而，支架较长或串联置入支架时还是应该进行高压后扩张，压力也不宜过高（12～14atm），以免增加无复流发生率。应当避免支架膨胀不完全和支架直径过小。血栓负荷重和为避免远端栓塞而低压释放是导致支架贴壁不良的两个因素。

最新证据表明，新一代DES（依维莫司或佐他莫司）的有效性和安全性优于BMS或第一代DES。

采用直接PCI常用的投照体位。一般采用两个投照体位从不同角度评估支架膨胀、病变覆盖是否完全。至少保证有一个投照体位的曝光时间要足够长，以便评价远端血流情况及是否有穿孔等并发症。

在没有PCI条件的医院，对于心源性休克或严重心力衰竭的STEMI患者，无论是否接受了溶栓治疗，也不论时间延迟情况，都应立即转运至有PCI条件的医院进行冠状动脉造影或PCI。溶栓失败或再闭塞的患者，有理由紧急转运至有PCI条件的医院行冠状动脉造影或补救性 PCI。临床判断溶栓成功并且病情稳定的 STEMI 患者，有理由在 24 小时内尽快转运至有 PCI 条件的医院行冠状动脉造影或即刻 PCI，但是应在溶栓后 2 ～ 3 小时内进行。

未及时接受直接 PCI 的 STEMI 患者，不论是否接受了溶栓治疗，符合以下任何一种情况时都应接受旨在进行血运重建的心导管和冠状动脉造影检查：①心源性休克或严重急性心力衰竭；②出院前无创缺血评估提示为中高危的患者；③存在自发或容易诱发的心绞痛。溶栓失败或溶栓后梗死相关动脉再闭塞时有理由尽快进行旨在实施血管重建的冠状动脉造影检查。临床溶栓成功且稳定的患者出院前尽快安排冠状动脉造影检查是适宜的，最好在 24 小时内，但不应该安排在溶栓开始后 2 ～ 3 小时内。

对于溶栓后或未接受再灌注治疗的 STEMI 患者，符合以下任何一种情况时应针对严重狭窄的梗死相关动脉实施延迟 PCI：①发病后出现心源性休克或严重急性心力衰竭；②出院前无创缺血评估提示为中高危的患者；③住院期间有自发或轻微体力活动诱发的心绞痛。以下情况有理由实施延迟 PCI：①溶栓失败或再闭塞，可以尽快实施 PCI；②溶栓后梗死相关动脉开通、病情稳定但是存在严重狭窄时，可以在 24 小时内尽快实施 PCI，但不应该安排在溶栓开始后 2 ～ 3 小时内。溶栓后梗死相关动脉开通、病情稳定但是存在严重狭窄的 STEMI 患者，24 小时后作为有创策略的一部分，可以考虑实施 PCI。对于发病超过 24 小时无症状、血流动力学和心电稳定、没有严重缺血证据的单支或双支病变 STEMI 患者，其梗死相关动脉完全闭塞时不应实施延迟 PCI。

【抗栓治疗】

抗栓治疗是整个急诊 PCI 围手术期非常重要的一环，包括抗血小板治疗（阿司匹林、氯吡格雷、替格瑞洛和糖蛋白Ⅱ b/Ⅲ a 受体拮抗剂）和抗凝治疗（普通肝素、低分子量肝素和比伐卢定）。

（1）阿司匹林　主要通过抑制血小板中血栓烷 A_2（TXA_2）的生成，来抑制血小板聚集并起到抗血栓形成的作用。大剂量（＞ 160mg）阿司匹林可以不可逆地抑制 TXA_2 的生成。阿司匹林口服后需要 2 个小时才能达到最大作用。即刻嚼服大剂量阿司匹林,几乎可以同时发挥抗血小板的作用。目前没有证据表明急诊状态下口服阿司匹林肠溶制剂,可以达到与应用非肠溶制剂同样的效果。因此,一旦诊断STEMI,如果没有用药禁忌证,应即刻嚼服 300mg 非肠溶制剂的阿司匹林。之后应当每日 75 ~ 100mg 长期口服。

(2)P_2Y_{12} 受体抑制剂 国内有替格瑞洛和氯吡格雷。替格瑞洛可逆性结合血小板的二磷酸腺苷受体从而抑制血小板聚集,可在 1 ~ 3 小时内达到最大血药浓度和最大抗血小板作用。氯吡格雷则不可逆抑制血小板的 P_2Y_{12} 受体从而抑制血小板聚集。氯吡格雷为前体药物,需肝脏细胞色素 P450 酶代谢形成活性代谢物,因此受基因多态性的影响。氯吡格雷用药后 6 个小时开始发挥其临床抗血栓作用。

相比氯吡格雷,替格瑞洛具有更强和快速抑制血小板的作用,且不受基因多态性的影响。STEMI 直接 PCI 患者应优先选用替格瑞洛,应给予负荷量替格瑞洛 180mg,以后 90mg/ 次,2 次 / 日,至少 12 个月;难以获得替格瑞洛时,应当给予氯吡格雷600mg 负荷量,以后 75mg/ 次,1 次 / 日,至少 12 个月。肾功能不全(肾小球滤过率< 60ml/min)患者无需调整 P_2Y_{12} 受体抑制剂用量。金属裸支架置入后至少 1 个月(除非患者发生出血的危险性增加,应当给予最小剂量 2 周)、雷帕霉素洗脱支架置入后 3 个月、紫杉醇洗脱支架置入后 6 个月,并且在没有高危出血危险的患者,理想的给药时间是 12 个月。在发生支架内亚急性血栓高危的患者(无保护的左主干、左主干分叉或仅存的冠状动脉通畅)或已发生支架血栓的患者优先给予替格瑞洛。可以考虑进行血小板聚集检查。如果证实血小板聚集抑制率< 50%,可以考虑将氯吡格雷剂量增加到每日 150mg。替格瑞洛禁忌用于既往出血性脑卒中或中重度肝脏疾病的患者。年龄大于 75 岁患者使用替格瑞洛应权衡出血风险。

(3)糖蛋白 Ⅱ b/ Ⅲ a 受体抑制剂 包括阿昔单抗、依替巴肽或替罗非班,可以有效地阻断纤维蛋白原和其他的黏附蛋白通过糖蛋白 Ⅱ b/ Ⅲ a 受体与毗邻的血小板结合。在有效的双联抗血小板及抗凝治疗情况下,不建议 STEMI 患者造影前常规应用 GP Ⅱ b/ Ⅲ a 受体拮抗剂。高危患者或造影提示血栓负荷重、未给予适当负荷量P_2Y_{12} 受体抑制剂的患者可静脉使用替罗非班或依替巴肽。直接 PCI 时,冠状动脉内注射替罗非班有助于减少无复流、改善心肌微循环灌注。

（4）**普通肝素**　普通肝素是一种经济、有效和有长期使用经验的抗凝药物，在我国已经得到广泛应用。然而，在我国急性心肌梗死患者中，相当比例的患者没有达到早期肝素化，因此应当强调在急诊室或到达导管室之前早期、足量使用普通肝素。急诊 PCI 造影时给予普通肝素冲击剂量 3000U/kg，介入操作时追加至 70 ～ 100U/kg。根据 ACT 追加剂量。应用 HemoTec 装置监测活化的凝血时间（activated clotting time，ACT），ACT 至少应 ＞ 250 ～ 350s，而使用 Hemochron 装置时 ACT 至少应 ＞ 300 ～ 350s。联合使用 GP Ⅱ b/ Ⅲ a 受体拮抗剂时，普通肝素剂量为 50 ～ 70U/kg，维持 ACT 200 ～ 250s。尽管应用普通肝素的剂量以及合理疗程尚无定论，但是，合理的治疗方案应该是静脉普通肝素治疗 48 小时，然后改为皮下应用肝素治疗。使用肝素期间应监测血小板计数，及时发现肝素诱导的血小板减少症（HIT）。

年龄 ＜ 75 岁的溶栓治疗患者，如果没有严重肾功能不全（血浆肌酐水平，男性 ＞ 2.5 mg/dl，女性 ＞ 2.0 mg/dl），低分子肝素可替代普通肝素作为辅助治疗用药。年龄 ＜ 75 岁的患者，依诺肝素 30mg 静脉注射，随后 1.0mg/kg 皮下注射 12 小时 1 次，直到出院。

（5）**比伐卢定**　是一种直接凝血酶抑制剂。对于 HIT 患者可以应用比伐卢定替代肝素。出血风险较高的患者也可以使用。静脉推注比伐卢定 0.75mg/kg，继而 1.75mg/（kg·h）静脉滴注（合用或不合用替罗非班），并维持至 PCI 后 3 ～ 4 小时，以减低急性支架血栓形成的风险。出血风险高的 STEMI 患者，单独使用比伐卢定可能优于联合使用普通肝素和 GP Ⅱ b/ Ⅲ a 受体拮抗剂。

（6）**磺达肝癸钠**　有增加导管内血栓形成的风险，不宜单独用作 PCI 时的抗凝选择。

冠状动脉无复流（no reflow）是指心外膜冠状动脉狭窄或闭塞被解除后心肌组织水平无灌注的现象。无复流现象也可发生于脑、肾脏、皮瓣组织，心肌无复流现象最早发现于 1966 年（猫心肌缺血再灌注模型），1985 年首次在溶栓患者中观察到人心肌无复流现象。从机制上讲无复流与罪犯病变部位血栓或斑块物质脱落导致的远端栓塞不同，其机制是微血管水平血流受阻和微循环功能障碍，有血小板或纤维蛋白聚集、微栓子形成、心肌和内皮细胞水肿、心肌内出血等现象，涉及炎症和缺血再灌注损伤等分子机制。有多种方法评价无复流，如示踪剂、ST 段回落率、造影 TIMI 血流分级、造影心肌染色分级、压力导丝测定、心肌声学造影、磁共振成像等。因此，无复流的发生率报道差异也较大。无复流的临床造影定义为：在没有心外膜动脉阻塞、夹层、痉挛或原位血栓形成情况下，冠脉血流的急剧减少。其中，TIMI 血流分级 0～1 级者为无复流，TIMI 血流分级 2 级也被称为慢血流。实际上，冠状动脉造影有时无法区分开远端栓塞和无复流现象。直接 PCI 时无复流的发生率明显高于择期 PCI，并增加远期死亡率。直接 PCI 术中发生无复流时可冠脉内推注（IC）血管扩张剂。常用血管扩张剂有：维拉帕米（100～200μg IC，总量可达 1000μg）、地尔硫卓（500～1000μg IC，总量可达 5000μg）、硝普钠（50～200μg IC，总量可达 1000μg）、尼可地尔（2～5mg）和腺苷（10～20μg 弹丸式注射，有研究提示腺苷 240μg IC 耐受性良好）。研究显示硝普钠、钙拮抗药和腺苷治疗无复流的效果没有明显差异，因此血管扩张剂可以任选上述任何一种，除腺苷外均应缓慢冠状动脉内推注，密切注意血压、心率的变化。血压较低时应严格控制药物推注剂量，可采用少量、多次推注的原则。钙拮抗药、腺苷常导致心率下降，可静脉推注阿托品和（或）多巴胺纠正。有报道冠脉内推注尼可地尔纠正无复流效果也较好。硝酸甘油治疗无复流效果较差。不过，硝酸甘油属于 PCI 术中常规备药，因此，可视血压情况先尝试冠状动脉内推注 50～200μg，也有助于鉴别是否有心外膜冠状动脉痉挛因素。冠脉内推注 GPI（如替罗非班 500～1000μg IC）也可能有助于缓解无复流。由于有时无法有效区分无复流或远端栓塞（两者也可能同时发生），血栓抽吸也可以作为一项重要的处置措施。

与直接 PCI 有关的并发症与择期 PCI 导致的并发症相似，但其发生率较高。介入手术并发症可以分为严重并发症（死亡、心肌梗死和卒中）和轻微并发症（一过性脑缺血发作、血管路径并发症、肾功能不全和对比剂不良反应）。其他特殊并发症包括冠状动脉栓塞、冠状动脉穿孔、心脏压塞和心律失常。综合分析 STEMI 直接 PCI 的结果显示其期短期死亡率为 7%。即使排除了心源性休克患者后，住院死亡率仍在 5% 左右。需要施行急诊 CABG 是 PCI 的潜在并发症。在支架时代 STEMI 患者的急诊 CABG 率为 0.4%。

心源性休克是 STEMI 合并住院死亡率的头号原因，死亡率高达 50% 以上。85%的休克病例诊断于 STEMI 开始治疗之后，但多数是 24 小时之内发生休克。血管重建是能够降低心源性休克死亡率的唯一治疗手段。虽然这类患者几乎全部都是采用 PCI完成血管重建治疗，但是经过选择的严重三支或左主干病变患者可以从急诊 CABG中获益。有严重多器官衰竭时，血管重建治疗可能无效并且没有指征。在老年患者，选择患者做血管重建治疗更为重要，但是在没有合并性疾病的患者中结果也较好，并且可以有存活受益。由于不转运的死亡率明显增高，因此没有 PCI 能力的医院应紧急转运患者到有 PCI 能力的医院进行血运重建。紧急血运重建的时间窗很宽，有研究显示可达心肌梗死后 54 小时和心源性休克后 18 小时。因此，STEMI 合并心源性休克或严重心功能不全的患者，不论时间延迟长短，均应进行直接 PCI。心源性休克患者的术前评估十分重要。心源性休克患者应当接受标准的药物治疗，包括阿司匹林、P_2Y_{12} 受体拮抗剂和抗凝。正性肌力药物和血管加压药物治疗能够提高灌注压。避免使用负性肌力药物和血管扩张剂。有关静脉使用糖蛋白 Ⅱb/Ⅲa 抑制剂是否可以获益，存在争议。

通常有必要对呼吸衰竭的患者实施气管插管和应用正性呼气末压的机械性通气。对心动过缓或高度房室传导阻滞的患者有指征置入临时起搏器。肺动脉导管检查可以提供有关应用并滴定正性肌力药物和血管加压药物剂量的信息。可以应用 IABP 或经皮左室辅助装置提供进一步的血流动力学支持，但是没有资料支持能够降低死亡率。

PCI 术中应当最大程度减少对比剂用量。左冠状动脉两个相互垂直位的血管造影像和右冠状动脉左前斜位血管造影像通常足以识别梗死相关动脉。虽然作为手术的一部分，多数接受血管重建治疗的患者会接受一个支架，但是支架术与球囊血管成形术比较的资料相互矛盾。没有资料比较心源性休克时选择金属裸支架与药物洗脱支架。然而，常常应用金属裸支架是因为往往不清楚急诊状态下长期双联抗血小板治疗的依从性。

在多支血管病变患者，对非梗死相关动脉施行血管重建治疗对于最大程度增加心肌灌注可能是必要的。作为可供选择的方法，在多支血管病变尤其是左主干病变患者，可以优先选择作为主要再灌注策略的急诊 CABG。对血管重建治疗无反应的顽固性心源性休克，可能要求更为强化的心脏支持——左室辅助装置或其他血流动力学装置，使得心肌恢复或在适合的患者后续施行心脏移植。

新版指南提出，应当考虑在 PPCI 同时或出院前分次处理严重狭窄（血管造影或 FFR 评估）。在心源性休克患者，应当在 PPCI 同时处理非罪犯病变。该要点已经成为目前的共识。问题是 PPCI 时评估非罪犯病变的生理学意义（即使使用 FFR）可能受 STEMI 时冠状动脉处于痉挛状态导致高估的影响。在 STEMI 合并多支严重病变拟采取一次性处理策略时要考虑患者的抗栓水平、病变血管的解剖结果和手术的复杂性，以及术者的经验和能力。

缓慢性心律失常（包括窦性心动过缓、窦性停搏、窦房阻滞、交界性心律和二度、三度房室传导阻滞）是 STEMI 右冠状动脉急性闭塞直接 PCI 中最常遇到的问题。缓慢性心律失常可以由窦房结缺血或迷走张力增高所致，高度房室阻滞通常是房室结缺血的结果。继发性心房与心室同步功能丧失，在右室功能障碍时可导致低血压和休克。无论是否出现右室心肌缺血或梗死，下壁心肌梗死患者常发生心动过缓和低血压，这可能是由于下后壁缺血刺激迷走传入的心脏抑制性反射所介导。这种作用在直接 PCI 后右冠状动脉出现再灌注时尤为明显。有些术者最常采用的处理方法是右心室临时起搏。但是，起搏电极在这类患者可诱发快速性心律失常，心室颤动发生率为 35.3%，起搏电极还有导致心脏穿孔风险（2%），应谨慎使用。直接 PCI 时静脉推注阿托品可以有效提高心率（其中部分恢复窦性心率，更加符合生理状况）并有助于维持血压，同时可以避免右心室起搏诱发的心室颤动和潜在的心脏穿孔风险。因此，静脉注射阿托品是处理直接 PCI 中缓慢性心律失常的首选措施。咳嗽也能刺激交感神经引起心跳加快，可嘱患者以咳嗽作为静脉推注阿托品起效前的过渡措施。此外，这类患者发生缓慢性心律失常的同时常伴有明显血压下降，可以静脉推注多巴胺 3～5mg，继之静脉泵入。同时，多巴胺也有提高患者心率的作用，但应注意多巴胺有潜在的致心律失常作用。当然，药物处理缓慢性心律失常效果不明显、血流动力学不能维持时应及时进行临时起搏。由于直接 PCI 术中进行颈内静脉、锁骨下静脉穿刺置入临时起搏电极的操作与 PCI 操作互相干扰，肝素化条件下颈内静脉、锁骨下静脉穿刺颈部或纵隔出血风险也增加，直接 PCI 术中应首选股静脉穿刺置入临时起搏电极。

STEMI 机械并发症：STEMI 后机械并发症时间上呈双峰分布，大多数在第一个 24 小时以内，其余发生在第一周以内。心脏破裂是 STEMI 主要的机械并发症，包括乳头肌断裂引起二尖瓣反流、室间隔穿孔和心脏游离壁破裂引起心脏压塞。STEMI 发生机械并发症多为外科手术指征。在就诊时至诊断性造影前应仔细查体，发现心脏杂音等提示室间隔穿孔或乳头肌断裂的线索时尽快行 UCG 检查明确诊断。室间隔穿孔患者血流动力学处于代偿期时应当置入 IABP 并尽早进行外科修补术。有病例报道称经皮封堵术可以用于室间隔穿孔的治疗，在手术量大的医学中心可能将会取代外科手术。发生游离壁破裂引起心脏压塞时，应当尽快进行心包穿刺引流和外科修补。左室游离壁破裂占心肌梗死患者住院死亡率的 15%。SHOCK 注册研究显示，左室游离壁破裂的患者无论是否进行外科修补术其死亡率相当。乳头肌断裂导致急性二尖瓣反流的患者，应当尽快进行外科缝合和血运重建。

有大约 1/3 下壁 STEMI 伴有右室心肌梗死，绝大多数右室心肌梗死病变位于右冠状动脉近段。所有下壁 STEMI 患者都应仔细寻找是否有右室梗死的证据。低血压、肺野清晰和颈静脉压增高是右室梗死的三联征。V_1 和 V_4R 导联 ST 段抬高 $\geq$ 1mm 是右室损伤最敏感的心电图表现。早期证据不明显时，经胸 UCG 可能有助于发现右室心肌梗死。治疗包括维护右室前负荷（视左心功能情况适当快速输注晶体或胶体液）、降低右室后负荷，必要时正性肌力药物和尽快再灌注治疗。应该避免使用硝酸酯类药物和利尿剂。右心室游离壁主要由右心室锐缘支供血，因此右室功能障碍程度与右心室锐缘支血流受损程度有关。事实上，直接 PCI 不能迅速恢复右室锐缘支血流与右室功能得不到恢复、持续低血压、低心排血量和死亡率增加都有关系。急性右室心肌梗死患者室性心律失常的发生率高，下壁合并右室心肌梗死患者发生死亡、休克和心律失常的危险性增加。这种高危险性与右室心肌本身受累有关，而与左室心肌损害范围无关。下壁心肌梗死 6 小时以内直接 PCI 可以提高合并右室心肌梗死患者的短期生存率。血流动力学有明显改变的右室心肌梗死死亡率较高，采用直接 PCI 可取得最佳效果。

直接 PCI 时应该系统治疗梗死相关动脉。直接 PCI 同期（即刻预防性）治疗非梗死相关动脉仍有争议。以下情况应该直接 PCI 时酌情处理非梗死相关动脉可以更为积极：①有多支严重病变但根据心电图等不能明确判断梗死相关动脉时；②心源性休克患者其非梗死相关动脉较大且有严重病变，对其进行 PCI 可能改善血流动力学状况时。

STEMI 后应用药物治疗不能够很快稳定病情的心源性休克患者，应该使用经皮血流动力学支持装置。在经过仔细选择的高危患者，可以择期插入适合的血流动力学支持装置作为 PCI 的一种辅助措施。IABP 已广泛应用于心源性休克患者的机械支持治疗。然而，IABP-SHOCK Ⅱ 研究结果对 IABP 的效果提出了挑战。该研究涉及598 例 AMI（包括 STEMI 和 NSTEMI）合并心源性休克接受早期血运重建的患者，其结果和 12 个月随访显示常规使用 IABP 并不降低 30 天和 1 年死亡率。不过，该研究也显示 IABP 没有增加严重出血、卒中和肢体缺血事件。经皮左心室辅助装置（Impella 或 TandemHeart）对于血流动力学的改善优于 IABP，但并没有降低死亡率和下肢缺血事件，其出血事件高于 IABP。Impella Recover LP 2.5 系统是经皮经 13 Fr 股动脉鞘插入一根 12.5 Fr 导管，横跨主动脉瓣至左心室，一个经轴向血液泵通过该导管提供高达 2.5 L/min 的血流。该系统已经应用于心源性休克患者和择期 PCI。已经在高危 PCI 患者对 Impella 2.5 系统的血流动力学效果进行了研究，证实了有益的左心室去负荷效果（降低舒张末压和室壁张力），左心室整体或收缩功能没有改变。一项试验在 20 例应用 Impella 2.5 系统接受高危 PCI 的患者得出结论，该装置安全、易于置入，有明显的血流动力学效果。欧洲注册研究包括了 144 例接受高危 PCI 的患者，结果安全、可行并且有潜在应用价值，因而提出需要进行随机对照试验。一项随机试验旨在证实 Impella 的 1 个月不良事件优于主动脉内气囊反搏术，结果由于分析中期研究结果显示无效而中止试验。TandemHeart 是一种左心房到主动脉的导管系统，包括一个能够提供高达 4L/min 血流的血液输出泵。该装置使用 21 Fr 导管经皮插入股静脉作为左心房经间隔路径，与放置在对侧股动脉并且定位于主动脉分叉处的 15 Fr 导管连接。然后，体外循环泵从左心房回输氧合的血液至动脉系统，因而去负荷左心室。在接受高危 PCI 的患者已经研究了血流动力学效应，显示了 TandemHeart 的临床效果。一项单中心 68 例患者应用 TandemHeart 或 Impella Recover 2.5 接受高危 PCI 的结果显示，成功率（＞90%）和血管并发症（7%）相当。此外，对于 STEMI 合并心源性休克在接受直接 PCI、最佳药物治疗和 IABP 支持仍无改善的情况下，可以使用体外膜肺氧合（ECMO）技术。

患者风险、血流动力学支持、容易应用/拔除、术者，以及导管室的专门知识，都是考虑应用这些装置的影响因素。由于装置需要插入大的导管，因此，血管损伤的风险和相关并发症是应用该装置必要性和选择的重要考虑。

STEMI 时需要 CABG 的情况较少见。由于 CABG 准备时间较长、STEMI 时外科手术风险较高，因此 STEMI 急性期 CABG 获益有限或不明确。STEMI 急性期应当行急诊 CABG 的 I 类指征包括：①直接 PCI 失败；②冠状动脉解剖不适合 PCI，但仍有持续或反复心肌缺血、心源性休克、严重心力衰竭或其他高危因素；③有需要外科修复的机械并发症（如室间隔穿孔、乳头肌断裂或游离壁破裂）。存在心源性休克并且适合 CABG 的患者，不考虑心肌梗死到休克发生的间隔时间和心肌梗死到 CABG 的时间。

【STEMI 急诊 CABG 的抗血小板停药问题】

I 类建议：①急诊 CABG 前不应停用阿司匹林；②体外循环 CABG 时，如有可能，停用氯吡格雷或替格瑞洛 24 小时以上；③急诊 CABG 前应停用短效 GPI（依替巴肽或替罗非班）至少 2～4 小时，停用阿西单抗至少 12 小时。

Ⅱb 类建议：①氯吡格雷或替格瑞洛服药 24 小时内可以考虑急诊不停跳 CABG，尤其是血管重建获益高于出血风险时；②氯吡格雷或替格瑞洛服用 5 天内或普拉格雷服用 7 天内可以考虑急诊 CABG，尤其是血管重建获益高于出血风险时。

第六章
住院期间和出院时的处理

第 1 节　冠状动脉监护病房 / 重症监护病房

再灌注治疗后应将 STEMI 患者转入可持续监测并有专业看护能力的冠心病监护病房、心脏重症监护病房或等同条件的病房。医护人员应熟悉 ACS、心律失常、心力衰竭、机械性循环支持、有创或无创血流动力学监测（动脉和肺动脉压力）、呼吸监测、机械通气和体温调控。监测病房应有能力处理患者的严重肾脏和肺部疾病。冠心病监护病房 / 心脏重症监护病房的组织、结构及标准参照 ESC 急性心血管治疗协会（Acute Cardiovascular Care Association，ACCA）标准文件。

第 2 节　监护

建议对所有患者 STEMI 发病后进行心电监测心律失常和 ST 段变化至少 24 小时。对于心律失常发生可能性中高危的患者（合并以下 1 种以上情况：血流动力学不稳定、严重心律失常、LVEF ＜ 40%、再灌注失败、其他主要冠状动脉存在严重狭窄或发生 PCI 并发症），应当进行长时间心电监测。进一步的心电监测取决于风险评估。患者转出冠心病监护病房 / 心脏重症监护病房或等同病房后可以进行心电遥测。患者在需要持续心电监测的窗口期进行转运时，应配置足够的训练有素的人力，以便应对致命性心律失常及心脏骤停。

第 3 节　离床活动

大多数患者建议早期活动（第 1 天），经桡动脉入径 PCI 有助于早期活动。对于有严重心肌损伤、心力衰竭、低血压和心律失常的患者，在心功能评估和临床状态稳定之前可以卧床休息。合并大面积心肌梗死和严重合并症的患者，取决于其症状和体能条件，有时需要延长卧床时间和限制体力活动。

第 4 节　住院时间

在冠心病监护病房 / 心脏重症监护病房和在院治疗的最佳时限取决于患者个体的基础情况、心脏风险、合并症、功能状态和社会支持情况（表 6-1）。再灌注治疗的成功和冠状动脉解剖情况评估的普及使 STEMI 后住院时间和 30 天的死亡率进一步缩短，提示早期出院与晚期心脏死亡率无关。多个研究显示，低危患者及时进行 PCI 和完全血运重建后第 2 天或第 3 天出院是安全的。可以采用简单标准（如 PAMI-Ⅱ 标准、ZeollePPCI 指数或其他标准）筛选 STEMI 后适合早期离院的患者。PAMI-Ⅱ 低危患者标准：年龄＜ 70 岁伴有 LVEF ＞ 45%、单支到双支血管病变或 PCI 成功，并且没有持续性心律失常。不过，住院时间短意味着患者宣教和二级预防时间有限。因此，这些患者离院后应接受心脏专科医师、社区医师或专业护士的定期随访，并尽快纳入院内或门诊的正规康复计划。

PPCI 成功后早期（即当天）可以常规转运至地方医院继续治疗。对于经过筛选的患者（如无进行性心肌缺血的症状体征、无心律失常、血流动力学稳定、不需要血管活性药物及机械支持和无进一步血运重建计划），转运至地方医院并在充分监测和监护下继续治疗是安全的。

表 6-1　住院调度问题

建议	建议类别	证据水平
建议所有参与 STEMI 患者救治的医院设立 CCU 或 ICCU，并能提供全方位的 STEMI 救治，包括针对缺血、严重心力衰竭、心律失常和常见并发症的治疗	I	C
转回指定的非 PCI 医院		
直接 PCI 成功后，应该考虑将部分患者（例如无心肌缺血、心律失常发作，循环稳定而不需要血管活性药物或机械辅助支持，并且不需要进一步早期血运重建治疗）当天转至非 PCI 医院	IIa	C
监测		
建议所有 STEMI 患者行心电监测至少 24 小时	I	C
CCU 住院时间		
建议再灌注治疗成功且无临床并发症患者在 CCU 或 ICCU 住院至少 24 小时，之后转至次级监测病床观察 24 ～ 48 小时	I	C
出院		
低危患者[a] 如果已安排了合理的早期康复和随访计划应考虑早期出院	IIa	A

注：CCU：冠心病监护病房；ICCU：重症心脏监护病房；PCI：经皮冠状动脉介入术治疗；STEMI：ST 段抬高型心肌梗死。

[a] 如 PAMI-II 标准：年龄＜ 70 岁、LVEF ＞ 45%、单支或双支病变、PCI 成功并且无持续性心律失常。

第 5 节　特殊患者

以下几类特殊人群应特殊对待。

1. 口服抗凝药物的患者

很多 STEMI 的患者既往服用口服抗凝药或者需要长期抗凝治疗。与单纯抗凝治疗相比，抗凝治疗联合双联抗血小板使出血风险增加 2 ～ 3 倍。

STEMI 发病时的处理：口服抗凝药是溶栓治疗的相对禁忌证。因此，口服抗凝药的 STEMI 患者不论时间延迟长短都应实施 PPCI 进行再灌注治疗。无需考虑患者末次口服抗凝药的时间，所有患者都应采用肠外抗凝。避免使用糖蛋白 II b/ III a 抑制剂。所有 STEMI 患者均建议服用负荷剂量的阿司匹林，P_2Y_{12} 抑制剂建议使用氯吡格雷（负荷剂量 600mg，于 PCI 术前或最迟 PCI 术中服用。不建议使用普拉格雷和替格瑞洛。长期抗凝药物在住院期间最好不要停用。建议同时服用质子泵抑制剂保护胃黏膜。

STEMI 后的处理：对有双联抗血小板治疗指征的患者（例如 STEMI 后），应当仔细评估是否继续服用口服抗凝药，有必须服用的证据时才继续使用。要同时考虑出血和缺血的风险。有相当多的危险因素既可以预测缺血也可以预测出血。CHA2DS2-VASC 评分[心力衰竭、高血压、年龄 ≥ 75 岁（2 分）、糖尿病、卒中（2 分）-血管疾病、年龄 65 ～ 74 岁和性别（女性）] 用于预测缺血事件风险，还有多种评分用于预测出血风险。

多数患者三联抗栓治疗（口服抗凝药、阿司匹林、氯吡格雷）应维持 6 个月，之后后再继续口服抗凝药联合阿司匹林或氯吡格雷 6 个月，1 年之后单用口服抗凝药。出血风险极其高危的 STEMI 患者三联抗栓治疗可以缩短至 1 个月，继续双联抗栓治疗（口服抗凝药联合阿司匹林或氯吡格雷）满 1 年后单用口服抗凝药。

应密切监测口服抗凝药的强度，维持国际标准化比值在建议范围的低限。使用非维生素 K 拮抗剂类口服抗凝药时，应当采用卒中预防的最低有效剂量，通常不建议使用低于药物说明剂量的方案。近期一项涉及 2124 例非瓣膜性房颤接受 PCI 置入支架患者（约 12%STEMI）的开放、随机、对照、多中心临床研究（PIONEER AF-PCI）比较了三种抗栓治疗方案的效果。三种方案分别为低剂量利伐沙班（15mg qd）+ 一种 P_2Y_{12} 抑制剂（93% 为氯吡格雷）12 个月、极低剂量利伐沙班（2.5mg bid）+DAPT（95% 为氯吡格雷）持续 1 个月、6 个月或 12 个月和标准剂量维生素 K 拮抗剂 +DAPT（96% 为氯吡格雷）1 个月、6 个月或 12 个月。研究显示，使用利伐沙班的两组主要安全性终点（TIMI 严重出血）发生率低于维生素 K 拮抗剂组。三组之间严重出血和输血事件没有差别。不过，这项研究评价缺血性事件如支架血栓或卒中的效力不足，因此卒中和（或）支架血栓高危患者应用三种抗栓方案的效果还不明确。

2. 老年患者

随着人口老龄化，预计老年患者中 STEMI 的发生率将逐渐增高。老年患者心肌梗死的症状往往不典型，容易发生误诊和治疗不及时。由于老年患者合并症较多，其接受再灌注治疗的比例低于年轻患者。此外，由于老年患者出血风险随着年龄增高、肾功能下降及合并症较多，因此其急性期治疗的出血和并发症风险特别高。观察性研究显示，老年患者频繁发生抗栓药物过量的情况，其机械并发症的风险也较高。

关键是要对症状表现不典型的老年患者保持心肌梗死的高度警惕性，遵照指南建议进行治疗以及采用特殊策略降低出血风险。具体包括注意抗栓药物剂量恰当，特别是与肾功能不全、体质虚弱或合并症的关系，尽可能使用桡动脉入路。对于老年患者而言，再灌注治疗尤其是 PPCI 没有年龄上限。

3. 肾功能不全

ACS 患者中 30% ～ 40% 存在肾功能不全 [估测肾小球滤过率 eGFR ＜ 30ml/（min·1.73m²）]。肾功能不全与预后不良和院内并发症风险增高相关。由于肾功能不全患者临床表现的特殊性（很少有胸痛和典型心电图表现），容易发生诊断不及时。

尽管对于 STEMI 患者不得不在获得肾功能评估的结果之前做出介入治疗的决策，尽快评估 eGFR 还是非常重要的。应当根据患者的肾功能选择抗栓药物的类型、剂量（表 6-2），以及造影剂用量。合并慢性肾病患者经常接受过量的抗栓药物并导致出血风险增加。因此，对于已知或估计肾功能下降的患者，同时使用几种抗栓药物应当避免或者适当减量。确保在 PPCI 期间和术后适当水化、限制对比剂用量和首选低渗对比剂是降低对比剂肾病风险的重要措施。

表 6-2　慢性肾病患者 STEMI 急性期抗栓药物的建议剂量

药物	肾功能正常或 CKD 1～3 期 [eGFR ≥ 30ml/（min·1.73m²）]	CKD 4 期 [15 ≤ eGFR < 30 ml/（min·1.73m²）]	CKD 5 期 [eGFR < 15 ml/（min·1.73m²）]
阿司匹林	负荷量 150～300mg 口服，维持量 75～100mg qd	不需调整剂量	不需调整剂量
氯吡格雷	负荷量 300～600mg 口服，维持量 75mg qd	不需调整剂量	无有效信息
替格瑞洛	负荷量 180mg 口服，维持量 90mg bid	不需调整剂量	不建议使用
普拉格雷	负荷量 60mg 口服，维持量 10mg qd	不需调整剂量	不建议使用
依诺肝素	1mg/kg 皮下注射 bid；> 75 岁人群，0.75mg/kg 皮下注射 bid	1mg/kg 皮下注射 qd	不建议使用
UFH	冠状动脉造影前：60～70IU/kg 负荷量静脉推注（最多 5000IU），随后静脉输注 [12～15IU/（kg·h），最多 1000IU/h]，目标 APTT 维持在正常值的 1.5～2.5 倍 PCI 期间：70～100IU/kg 静脉推注（联合使用糖蛋白 Ⅱ b/Ⅲ a 抑制剂时剂量为 50～70IU/kg）	不需调整剂量	不需调整剂量
磺达肝癸钠	2.5mg 皮下注射 qd	若 eGFR < 20 ml/（min·1.73m²）或者血液透析者不建议使用	不建议使用
比伐卢定	0.75mg/kg 负荷量静脉推注，继之以 1.75mg/（kg·h）静脉输注。如果 eGFR 在 30～60ml/（min·1.73m²）之间则减量至 1.4mg/（kg·h）	不建议使用	不建议使用
阿昔单抗	0.25mg/kg 负荷量静脉推注，继之以 0.125μg/（kg·min）静脉输注（最多 100μg/min）	谨慎考虑出血风险	谨慎考虑出血风险

药物	肾功能正常或 CKD 1 ～ 3 期 [eGFR ≥ 30ml/（min · 1.73m²）]	CKD 4 期 [15 ≤ eGFR < 30 ml/（min · 1.73m²）]	CKD 5 期 [eGFR < 15 ml/（min · 1.73m²）]
依替巴肽	180μg/kg 负荷量静脉推注 [a]，继之以 2.0μg/（kg·min）静脉输注至 18 小时。若 eGFR < 50ml/（min · 1.73m²）则减量至 1.0μg/（kg·min）	不建议使用	不建议使用
替罗非班	25μg/kg 负荷量静脉推注，继之以 0.15μg/（kg·min）静脉输注	输注剂量减半	不建议使用

注：APTT：部分活化凝血活酶时间；CKD：慢性肾病；eGFR：估计的肾小球滤过率；UFH：普通肝素。
[a] 直接 PCI 时使用则需双倍负荷量。

4. 未灌注治疗的患者

由于特殊原因（如长时间延迟）未能在建议时间（最初 12 小时）内接受再灌注治疗的患者，应立即对其评估是否存在临床、血流动力学或心电不稳定情况。存在进行性心肌缺血、心力衰竭、血流动力学不稳定或威胁生命的心律失常的症状或体征时，应实施 PPCI。对于发病 12 ～ 48 小时病情稳定没有症状的患者，也应考虑实施 PPCI。此后，应考虑通过无创检查评价残留的心肌缺血或心肌存活情况，来决定延迟介入治疗或择期冠状动脉造影检查。然而，由于晚期并发症的风险增加，对于发病超过 48 小时梗死相关动脉完全闭塞的患者，不建议常规 PCI 治疗（图 6-1）。建议对所有患者早期进行超声心动图检查评价 LVEF。药物治疗应包括 DAPT、抗凝和二级预防。实施 PCI 的患者首选替格瑞洛或普拉格雷。未行 PCI 的患者建议氯吡格雷。冠状动脉血运重建前或出院前抗凝治疗首选使用磺达肝癸钠。应当强调，没有及时接受再灌注治疗的患者和及时接受再灌注治疗的患者一样，应当予以相同的二级预防治疗方案。

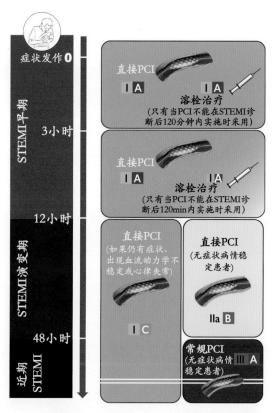

图 6-1 根据发病时间选择 IRA 再灌注治疗策略

注：对于早期就诊的患者（发病后 3 小时以内来诊断 STEMI），再灌注策略应该选择直接 PCI。若估计从 STEMI 诊断到 PCI 再灌注治疗时间＞120 分钟则应立即溶栓治疗。对于 3～12 小时内急诊的患者，就诊越晚就越应该考虑行直接 PCI；同时，就诊时间越晚就越不倾向于考虑溶栓治疗。对于 STEMI 进展期（发病 12～48 小时）患者，应该考虑常规直接 PCI 策略（急诊冠状动脉造影并在有指征时 PCI）。发病 48 小时后（近期 STEMI）的患者应该考虑进行冠状动脉造影，但不推荐对完全闭塞的 IRA 行常规 PCI。不论发病时间长短，如果患者有提示进行性缺血的症状、血流动力学不稳定或威胁生命的心律失常，都应实施直接 PCI 策略。

5. 糖尿病患者

与没有糖尿病患者相比，糖尿病患者更多表现为不典型的胸痛，从而更容易发生治疗延迟。糖尿病患者动脉粥样硬化病变也更为弥漫。尽管糖尿病患者的死亡和并发症（包括 PCI 后再次血运重建）风险高于没有糖尿病的患者，两者的抗栓和再灌注治疗方案没有区别。研究一致显示，糖尿病患者服用更强的 P_2Y_{12} 受体抑制剂（普拉格雷和替格瑞洛）较服用氯吡格雷获益大，更能降低绝对风险。不论既往是否有糖尿病或高血糖症，建议对所有 STEMI 患者和糖尿病患者测定血糖水平，并对糖尿病和高血糖症患者的血糖进行频繁监测。对重症患者进行强化胰岛素治疗时发生低血糖相关事件的概率升高。对于 STEMI 患者尚缺乏强有力的证据指导最佳血糖控制方案（如治疗阈值和血糖指标），严密而不苛刻的血糖控制似乎是最好的方案。在急性期，可以控制血糖（如维持血糖浓度≤ 11.0mmol/L 或 200mg/dl）但绝对避免发生低血糖。应用二甲双胍和（或）钠葡萄糖协同转运子 2（SGLT2）抑制剂的患者，建议监测 eGFR 以评估肾功能不全的风险。高血糖的管理见表 6–3。

表 6–3　高血糖的管理

建议	建议类别	证据水平
建议所有患者在进行初步评估时测量血糖水平，对于已知糖尿病或高血糖（血糖水平≥ 11.1mmol/L 或 200mg/dl）的患者定期监测血糖水平	I	C
服用二甲双胍和(或)钠 – 葡萄糖协同转运蛋白2（SGLT2）抑制剂的患者，建议在冠状动脉造影或 PCI 后至少 3 天内严密监测肾功能 [a]	I	C
血糖水平＞ 10mmol/L（＞ 180mg/dl）的 ACS 患者应该考虑降糖治疗，但应避免低血糖发作（血糖≤ 3.9mmol/L 或≤ 70mg/dl）	II a	C
合并晚期心血管疾病、高龄、长期糖尿病和其他并发症的 STEMI 急性期患者，血糖控制不应该太严格	II a	C

注：[a] 可以考虑在冠脉术后短期停用二甲双胍。

第 6 节　风险评估

1. 临床风险评估

对所有 STEMI 患者均应早期进行短期风险评估。包括心肌损伤范围、再灌注是否成功和是否有不良事件的高危临床指标（包括老年、快速心率、低血压、Killip 分级＞ 1、前壁心肌梗死、既往心肌梗死病史、首诊血肌酐升高、心力衰竭病史或外周动脉疾病）。目前已经建立了几个基于再灌注治疗前易于获得的急性期指标的评分系统。GRACE 评分建议用于风险的评估和校正。此外，对所有患者出院前都应进行远期风险评估，包括 LVEF、冠状动脉病变严重程度和冠状动脉血运重建的完全性、残余心肌缺血、住院期间并发症，以及代谢风险标志物的水平（包括总胆固醇、低密度脂蛋白胆固醇、高密度脂蛋白胆固醇、空腹甘油三酯、血浆血糖及肾功能）。由于心肌梗死后最初几天 LDL-C 水平有下降趋势，入院时应当尽早测定其水平。

没有接受成功再灌注治疗的患者早期并发症及死亡的风险较高。这些患者应予以评估残余缺血并在有条件的情况下评估心肌存活。因为事件发生风险随时间推移而下降，应进行早期风险评估。

2. 无创影像检查与风险分层

左室功能不全是影响预后的重要因素，建议所有 STEMI 患者出院前评估 LVEF。建议对心脏骤停、心源性休克、血流动力学不稳定、怀疑机械并发症或者不能确诊 STEMI 的患者行急诊心脏超声检查。建议 PPCI 后常规行超声心动图检查评估静息状态左心室、右心室功能和瓣膜功能，检查有无梗死后机械并发症及左室血栓形成。通常超声心动图可以满足以上需求。但是，有些病例超声心动图效果不清楚或不能确诊，此时心脏磁共振可能是一项理想的检查方法。对于多支血管病变仅处理了梗死相关动脉或者迟发 STEMI 患者，评估残余心肌缺血或心肌存活可以获益（表 6-4）。针对多支病变非梗死相关动脉病变的处理讨论参见第五章。患者心肌梗死急性事件结束数天后再发心绞痛或记录到心肌缺血并证明有大面积心肌存活时，倾向于择期对闭塞的梗死相关动脉进行血运重建。不过，这一策略目前还存在争议。

评估残余心肌缺血和心肌存活的时机和最佳影像技术（超声心动图、SPECT、心脏磁共振或 PET）还未确立，同时也取决于所在机构的设备和经验。最为广泛采用和深入研究的评估方法是负荷超声心动图和 SPECT（两者均结合运动或药物负荷），PET 和心脏磁共振也具有同等指征。不过，心肌梗死后患者由于存在室壁运动异常，应用超声心动图评价残余心肌缺血时面临一定挑战。延迟钆增强心脏磁共振技术在评估心肌瘢痕组织的透壁程度方面诊断精确性较高，但是检测存活心肌和预测室壁

表 6-4　ST 段抬高型心肌梗死患者影像学检查和负荷试验的适应证

建议	建议类别	证据水平
就诊时		
心源性休克和（或）血流动力学不稳定或怀疑合并机械并发症患者，建议在不延误冠状动脉造影前提下行急诊心脏超声检查	I	C
若诊断不明确，建议在冠状动脉造影前行急诊心脏超声检查	IIa	C
不建议进行延误急诊冠状动脉造影的常规行心脏超声检查	III	C
不建议行冠状动脉 CT 血管成像	III	C
住院期间（直接 PCI 术后）		
建议所有患者常规行心脏超声检查，以评估静息下左右心室功能、早期发现心肌梗死后机械并发症，以及排除左心室血栓形成	I	B
建议血流动力学不稳定患者进行行急诊心脏超声检查	I	C
若心脏超声结果不清晰或无法明确诊断时，应该考虑行其他影像学检查（建议行心脏磁共振检查）	IIa	C
可以考虑为患者（包括多支病变患者）进行负荷超声心动图、心脏磁共振、SPECT 或 PET 等任一检查，以评估有无心肌缺血及心肌活力	IIb	C
出院后		
出院前 LVEF ≤ 40% 的患者，建议在全血运重建和强化药物治疗基础上于心肌梗死后 6～12 周复查心脏超声，以评估是否需要置入 ICD 进行一级预防	I	C
心脏超声检查结果不清晰或无法明确诊断时，应该考虑其他影像学检查评估左心室功能（首选心脏磁共振检查）	IIa	C

注：ICD：置入式心律转复除颤器；PET：正电子发射计算机断层成像；SPECT：单光子发射计算机断层成像。

运动恢复的能力并不优于其他技术。延迟钆增强心脏磁共振检测到无功能存活心肌是缺血性左室功能不全患者死亡率的独立预测因子。

新近研究显示，变薄的室壁当瘢痕组织负荷有限时，血运重建后其收缩力和室壁厚度可以获得改善。这一结果提示了心肌存活的重要性和血运重建改善预后的作用。PET 也是具有高分辨率的一项技术，但是成本和可及性限制了其应用。一项采用 PET 技术的随机对照临床试验显示，患者存在大量无功能但是存活的心肌时接受血运重建可以获益，可以改善局部和整体的收缩功能、症状、活动耐力及远期预后。荟萃分析也显示存活心肌血运重建与生存率改善之间具有相关性。

对于出院前 LVEF ≤ 40% 的患者，建议在完全血运重建和强化药物治疗 6 ~ 12 周内再次测定 LVEF，以评价是否需要置入埋藏式心律转复除颤器进行一级预防。其他可以通过无创影像技术测定并且可以作为临床试验终点的参数包括：①梗死面积（心脏磁共振 、SPECT 和 PET）；②缺血心肌（SPECT 和心脏磁共振）；③微血管阻塞（心脏磁共振）；④心肌内出血（心脏磁共振）。其中，梗死范围和微血管阻塞是 STEMI 存活患者远期死亡和心力衰竭的预测因素。

⊕ | 评　注

本章主要讨论了 STEMI 患者入院后监护、住院时间、特殊患者和出院前风险评估。

STEMI 患者入院后的主要风险是发生心律失常、心力衰竭和机械性并发症，因此，对监护场所和相关医务人员提出了较高的要求。然而，国内许多基层医院缺乏必要的设备和受过专门训练的人员，因此需要按照指南的要求加大这些方面的投入。

对于接受急诊 PCI 并且没有并发症的 STEMI 患者，通常在监护病房观察 2 ~ 3 天后转入普通病房，继续观察 2 ~ 3 天后可以出院。然而，由于国内社区医疗的不完善，STEMI 患者通常在监护病房和普通病房的住院时间更长。重症患者的住院时间内取决于患者个体的基础情况、心脏风险、合并症、功能状态和出院后所能获得的医疗服务情况。

特殊患者包括口服抗凝药物的患者、老年患者、肾功能不全患者、未接受再灌注治疗的患者和糖尿病患者。对于口服抗凝药物并且接受了急诊 PCI 的患者，往往需要应用三联抗栓治疗，即 DAPT 联合一种口服抗凝药物。然而，虽然 DAPT 能够有效预防 PCI 后的支架血栓形成，但是不能有效降低心房颤动、心脏机械瓣置换术后和静脉血栓性疾病栓子脱落导致的栓塞风险。相反，单纯口服抗凝治疗对降低栓子脱落引起的栓塞风险有效，但是不能预防 PCI 后的支架血栓。三联抗栓治疗可以兼顾两者，但是出血风险成倍增高。因此，如何兼顾两者，同时最大程度降低出血风险，是临床面临的一个重要问题。临床研究中老年患者的年龄界限为 75 岁，而临床实践中往往缺乏明确的定义。老年患者的风险主要是合并肾功能损害和其他合并症，因此在各种风险评估中老年是一项独立的预测因素。合并肾功能不全患者面临的最主要问题是抗栓治疗导致的出血和对比剂相关的肾功能损害。对于未接受再灌注治疗的患者要进一步评估风险，采取积极的治疗。糖尿病患者往往胸痛表现不典型，动脉粥样硬化广泛和容易发生肾功能损害，临床预后更差。注意到这些特殊患者面临的主要风险，对于制订个体化治疗策略十分重要。

出院前风险评估包括临床评估和借助心脏超声、MRI 和（或）核素成像的评估。指南要求完成出院前风险评估，为患者制订出院后的个体方案。遗憾的是国内很少有医院能够这么做，应当引起重视。影像检查对于患者的鉴别诊断、功能评估和指导治疗非常重要。然而，不必要的左心室造影评估心功能、频繁拍摄胸片来评估肺水肿状态，以及反复进行不必要的 CT 检查，一方面会带来放射损伤的风险，另一方面会增加不必要的成本。心脏超声检查是一项无创、花费较少、易行和准确的心脏评估手段，已经广泛应用。每个病房应当配备便携式心脏超声仪，同时要求所有心脏科医师掌握检查技术和判读能力。

第七章

ST 段抬高型心肌梗死的长期治疗

第 1 节 生活方式干预和危险因素控制

主要的生活方式干预包括戒烟、强化血压控制、饮食建议和控制体重，并鼓励锻炼身体（表 7-1）。可从 ESC 预防指南获得详细的建议。住院期间实施二级预防的时间是有限的，心脏专科医师和全科医师，尤其专科康复护士、药剂师、营养师和理疗师之间的紧密合作非常重要。生活习惯是不容易改变的，并且这些改变的实施和维持是一个长期的过程。

1. 戒烟

吸烟有很强的致血栓前作用，戒烟可能是成本效益最高的二级预防措施。应当在住院期间开始戒烟干预，并且在出院后的随访期间继续。一项涉及 20 项观察性研究的荟萃分析（12 603 例）显示，烟有益，戒烟使冠心病包括心肌梗死患者死亡率降低 36%。

冠心病患者继续或重新开始吸烟的数量显著，说明了吸烟习惯的成瘾性。有强烈的证据支持进行短期干预戒烟，即结合行为支持和药物疗法（包括尼古丁替代疗法、安非他酮和伐尼克兰）。电子香烟也可以帮助实现戒烟。两项随机临床试验的荟萃分析（662 例）显示，与安慰剂相比，应用含有尼古丁的电子香烟的患者有较高的戒烟率或较低的再吸烟率。

2. 饮食，饮酒和体重控制

目前的预防指南建议：①地中海饮食，包括摄入的饱和脂肪不超过总能量的10%，通过摄入多元不饱和脂肪酸替代，并尽可能少摄入反式脂肪酸；②每日盐摄入量＜5g；③每日30～45g膳食纤维；④每日≥200g水果和200g蔬菜；⑤每周1～2次鱼类（尤其是油性鱼类）；⑥每日30g无盐坚果；⑦限制酒精摄入量[男性每日最多2杯(20g酒精)和女性最多1杯]；⑧不建议摄入含糖饮料。不建议戒酒者适量饮酒。

与健康体重（体重指数20～25kg/m²）相比，超重和肥胖（体重指数≥25kg/m²）与全因死亡率升高相关。腹型肥胖尤其有害，减重对控制心血管疾病危险因素有益。因此，建议所有人包括STEMI患者，保持健康体重或减重。然而，目前还没有证实减重本身能降低死亡率。

3. 运动心脏康复

所有急性心肌梗死患者应参与基于运动的心脏康复计划，并且要考虑年龄、梗死前的活动水平和体力限制。一项心脏康复计划最好包括运动训练、改变危险因素、教育、压力处理和心理支持。一项大规模荟萃分析表明，作为冠状动脉疾病患者心脏康复方案的一部分，运动可使心源性死亡率降低22%。心脏康复的好处可能是通过运动训练的直接生理效应、对危险因素的控制、生活方式和情绪心脏康复的效果来实现的。在住院时间短的背景下，心脏康复的另一个好处是能够保障STEMI后根据患者的实际情况对关键的循证学治疗方案进行监测和调整。目前，大多数康复训练为持续8～24周的门诊项目。

4. 恢复活动

急性心肌梗死后重返工作是一项重要的康复指标。年轻女性不返回工作岗位的风险尤其高，有证据表明女性心肌梗死后康复情况比同龄男性差。应根据左心室功能、血运重建和心率控制情况，以及工作特点制定个体化决策。长期病假通常无益，出院后应鼓励进行轻至中度体力活动。早期可恢复与体能相适应的性生活。

限制航空旅行的数据有限，包括在国外发生心肌梗死后的患者回国。与临床状况相关的因素及旅程长短、是否有人陪同和焦虑程度也发挥着作用。完全血运重建不伴有并发症并且 LVEF ＞ 40% 的心肌梗死患者风险较低，出院第 3 天后旅行认为是安全的。复杂的 STEMI 患者，包括伴有心力衰竭、LVEF ＜ 40%、残余缺血和心律失常情况，旅行应推迟到病情稳定之后。

5. 控制血压

高血压是 STEMI 患者一个常见的危险因素，因此应控制好血压。除了生活方式的改变（包括减少食盐的摄入量、增加体力活动和减轻体重），还应当开始药物治疗并控制收缩压目标值＜ 140mmHg。老年和体弱患者的目标可以宽松些，而对于非常高危且可耐受多种降压药物联合降压的患者，应当考虑收缩压目标值＜ 120mmHg。虽然已证明这样做非常有效，如果不坚持生活方式干预和药物治疗可以影响治疗的效果。

6. 治疗依从性

治疗依从性差是实现最佳治疗目标的重要障碍，并与不良结果相关。急性心肌梗死后患者门诊随访延迟导致短期和长期药物治疗依从性不佳。一项涉及 376 162 例患者的荟萃分析显示，随访 2 年时患者坚持应用心血管药物的比例推测为 57%。

一般认为，依从性是由社会经济、药物、环境、医疗制度和患者因素的相互作用决定的。一种改善依从性的策略是使用由主要降低心血管风险的药物植被的固定剂量复合剂或复方制剂，每日 1 次给药。唯一的针对心肌梗死后患者的研究是最近的 FOCUS(Fixed-Dose Combination Drug for Secondary Cardiovascular Prevention) Ⅱ期研究，该研究将 695 例心肌梗死后患者随机分为接受常规治疗组和复方制剂 [包括阿司匹林、一种血管紧张素转换酶抑制剂 （ angiotensin-converting enzyme inhibitor， ACEI ）和一种他汀] 治疗组。结果显示，与常规治疗组相比，平均随访 9 个月时复方制剂治疗组依从性改善。还需要大样本量研究进一步证实其在二级预防中的临床获益。

虽然已经确定低依从性是一个普遍存在的问题，但是医护人员和患者应当意识到这一挑战，通过提供明确的信息和简化治疗方案使医患沟通优化，做到共同决策并重复进行监测和反馈。

表 7-1　ST 段抬高型心肌梗死之后的生活方式

建议	建议类别	证据水平
建议确定患者是否吸烟。反复建议吸烟患者戒烟，通过随访支持、尼古丁替代治疗、伐尼克兰和安非他酮等方法单用或联用帮助其戒烟	I	A
建议患者参与心脏康复治疗	I	A
建议参与 STEMI 患者诊疗的医院为吸烟患者制定戒烟计划	I	C
可以考虑使用复方制剂和联合治疗方案增加患者对药物治疗的依从性	Ⅱb	B

<h1 style="text-align:center">第 2 节　抗栓治疗</h1>

这部分内容在同期发表的 ESC DAPT 指南更新版中有更详细叙述。

1. 阿司匹林

建议所有 STEMI 患者长期应用阿司匹林维持治疗（表 7-2）。CURRENT-OASIS 7 随机研究未能证明低剂量（75 ～ 100mg/d）和高剂量（300 ～ 325mg/d）的阿司匹林治疗 30 天后临床结果有差异。不过，低剂量组的胃肠道出血较少。以前的荟萃分析未能证明高于 100mg 的维持方案使患者获益，并且出血风险增加。建议采用低剂量维持量（75 ～ 100mg）进行长期预防。有阿司匹林过敏史的患者可以进行脱敏治疗后继续长期服用。真正不耐受阿司匹林的患者长期二级预防应服用氯吡格雷单药治疗（75mg/d）。目前正在进行使用替格瑞洛单药治疗替代阿司匹林进行二级预防的研究，在此还不能提出建议。

2. 双联抗血小板治疗和联合抗栓治疗的持续时间

（1）建议 PPCI 的 STEMI 患者 DAPT（联用阿司匹林和一种 P_2Y_{12} 受体抑制剂如普拉格雷、替格瑞洛或氯吡格雷）至 12 个月。溶栓后行 PCI 的 STEMI 患者也建议服用 DAPT 至 12 个月。对于溶栓后未行 PCI 和没有接受再灌注治疗的患者，建议 DAPT 1 个月并且应当考虑延长至 12 个月。

基于主要大规模研究的结果和专家共识，以前的指南建议 ACS 后 DAPT 持续时间 12 个月。不过，这一方案受到多个研究结果的挑战。这些研究包括了因不同临床适应证接受药物洗脱支架的患者，对比了 DAPT 12 个月与更短或更长时间 DAPT 治疗的效果。结果显示 DAPT 治疗持续时间要个体化，应根据出血和缺血风险决定，其是使用超过 12 个月时。

迄今为止，还没有专门的研究评估高出血风险患者最佳的 DAPT 维持时间。多个研究显示将 DAPT 从 12 个月（或更长）缩短至 6 个月可以降低严重出血并发症的风险，而缺血事件无明显增加。纳入 2013 例患者（其中 33% 为 STEMI）的 PRIDIGY（PROlonging Dual Antiplatelet Treatment After Grading stent-induced Intimal hyperplasia study）研究显示，CRUSADE 出血评分＞40 的高出血风险患者服用 DAPT 24 个月其严重出血和输血的绝对风险高于服用 6 个月，并且没有缺血获益。而在 CRUSADE（Can Rapid risk stratification of Unstable angina patients Suppress Adverse outcomes with Early implementation of the ACC/AHA guidelines）出血评分≤40 的患者中则没有观察到这种倾向。

有 2 项研究表明，超过 12 个月 DAPT 治疗可以降低非致死性缺血事件。DAPT 研究评估了延长氯吡格雷或普拉格雷超过 12 个月的获益，但该研究中只有 10% 的 STEMI 患者。目前没有将氯吡格雷或普拉格雷治疗时间从 12 个月延长至 30 个月带来获益的数据。因此，对于使用氯吡格雷或普拉格雷超过 1 年，没有正式的建议。

PEGASUS-TIMI 54 研究（Prior Heart Attack Using Ticagrelor Compared to Placebo on a Background of Aspirin-Thrombolysis in Myocardial Infarction 54）评估使用替格瑞洛超过 12 个月的获益，比较了在过去 1～3 年内发生过心肌梗死且高风险的患者在阿司匹林基础上使用两种剂量替格瑞洛（60mg 和 90mg，bid）和安慰剂的疗效。研究显示，与安慰剂相比，替格瑞洛 90mg 组（*HR*=0.85，95%*CI*：0.75～0.96；*P*=0.008）和

60mg 组（$HR=0.84$，$95\%CI$：$0.74 \sim 0.95$；$P=0.004$）的 MACE 都降低。替格瑞洛组汇总后与安慰剂组比较总死亡率没有差异，但心血管死亡率有轻微下降（$HR=0.85$，$95\%CI$：$0.71 \sim 1.00$；$P=0.06$）趋势，与非致死性事件率下降一致。与安慰剂组（阿司匹林单药治疗）相比，60mg 剂量替格瑞洛组的卒中发生率显著降低（$HR=0.75$，$95\%CI$：$0.57 \sim 0.98$；$P=0.03$）。两种剂量替格瑞洛组的出血发生率都明显升高（60mg 和 90mg 替格瑞洛组分别为：$HR=2.32$，$95\%CI$：$1.68 \sim 3.21$；$P < 0.001$，$HR=2.69$，$95\%CI$：$1.96 \sim 3.70$；$P < 0.001$）。监管机构已批准了 60mg 替格瑞洛方案用于心肌梗死后 1 年以上患者的治疗。亚组分析显示 STEMI 与 NSTEMI 患者用药效果一致。

根据现有的数据，可以考虑在可耐受 DAPT、没有出血并发症并且有一项缺血事件危险因素的患者，以阿司匹林加替格瑞洛 60mg bid 的形式延长 DAPT 超过 1 年（最多 3 年）。

（2）建议溶栓后可以选择氯吡格雷作为 P_2Y_{12} 受体抑制剂。强效 P_2Y_{12} 受体抑制剂在溶栓治疗患者中的有效性还没有得到充分评价，安全性（如出血并发症）也不明确。然而，溶栓后接受 PCI 的患者在经过一个安全期（姑且认为 48 小时）后，没有生物学背景理由认为强效的 P_2Y_{12} 受体抑制剂会增加风险，也不能断定不会发挥像在 PPCI 人群中那样优于氯吡格雷的效果。

（3）建议对有胃肠道出血病史的患者应用质子泵抑制剂保护胃黏膜。有多种出血危险因素 [如高龄、合并应用抗凝药、类固醇或非甾体类抗炎药（包括高剂量的阿司匹林）和幽门螺杆菌感染] 的患者也适合使用质子泵抑制剂。质子泵抑制剂对替格瑞洛或普拉格雷的药代动力学没有影响。同时，没有明确的证据显示一些质子泵抑制剂对氯吡格雷的药代动力学影响具有临床意义。

ATLAS ACS 2-TIMI 51 研究（Acute Coronary Syndrome-Thrombolysis In Myocardial Infarction 51 ）（15 526 例，50% 为 STEMI）评价了 ACS 后患者在阿司匹林和氯吡格雷基础上联用利伐沙班（一种 X a 因子拮抗剂）的效果。平均随访 13 个月的结果显示，低剂量的利伐沙班（2.5mg bid）降低心血管死亡、心肌梗死或卒中的复合主要终点和全因死亡率。此外，支架血栓形成减少 1/3。然而，非 CABG 相关的严重出血和颅内出血发生率增加 3 倍。重要的是高剂量利伐沙班（5mg bid）没有降低心血管死亡率或任意原因死亡率，但出血风险明显升高。基于 ATLAS ACS 2–TIMI 51 研究的结果，STEMI 后出血风险低的患者，在服用阿司匹林和氯吡格雷的基础上可以有选择的联合应用低剂量利伐沙班（2.5mg）。

表 7-2 ST 段抬高型心肌梗死之后的维持抗栓策略

建议	建议类别	证据水平
建议低剂量阿司匹林（75 ～ 100mg）抗血小板治疗	I	A
除非有禁忌证（如高危出血风险），建议 PCI 术后 DAPT 方案 12 个月，采用阿司匹林联合替格瑞洛或普拉格雷（普拉格雷或替格瑞洛没药或对其有禁忌证时使用氯吡格雷）	I	A
有高危胃肠道出血风险患者建议 PPI 联合 DAPT 治疗 [a]	I	B
有口服抗凝治疗指征的患者，建议口服抗凝药联合抗血小板治疗	I	C
有高危严重出血风险患者，可以考虑 P_2Y_{12} 受体抑制剂服用 6 月后停药	IIa	B
置入支架的 STEMI 患者有口服抗凝指征时，应该考虑三联治疗 [b]1 ～ 6 个月（权衡再发冠状动脉事件和出血事件风险）	IIa	C
除非有禁忌证（如高危出血风险），未行 PCI 的患者应该考虑 DAPT 治疗 12 个月	IIa	C
有左心室血栓患者，在影像学复查结果指导下给予抗凝治疗不超过 6 个月	IIa	C
可耐受 DAPT 且无出血并发症的缺血高风险患者 [c]，可以考虑采用最大剂量阿司匹林基础上联合替格瑞洛 60mg bid 的 DAPT 方案 12 个月以上至不超过 3 年	IIb	B
服用阿司匹林联合氯吡格雷治疗的低出血风险患者，可以考虑使用低剂量利伐沙班（2.5mg bid）	IIb	B
不建议替格瑞洛或普拉格雷联合阿司匹林及口服抗凝药作为三联抗栓方案	III	C

注：PPI：质子泵抑制剂。

[a] 胃肠道出血史，抗凝药物治疗，长期使用非甾体抗炎药或糖皮质激素，以及至少具有以下 2 项：≥ 65 岁、呼吸困难、胃食管反流病、幽门螺杆菌感染和长期饮酒。

[b] 指抗凝、阿司匹林和氯吡格雷。

[c] 定义为 ≥ 50 岁和至少具有以下 1 项：≥ 65 岁、糖尿病药物治疗、自发性急性心肌梗死病史、冠心病多支病变、慢性肾功能不全 [eGFR ＜ 60ml/（min·1.73m²）]。

TRA 2P-TIMI 50 研究（Thrombin Receptor Antagonist in Secondary Prevention of Atherothrombotic Ischemic Events-Thrombolysis In Myocardial Infarction 50）评价了凝血酶受体抑制剂的效果。26 449 例有心肌梗死、缺血性卒中或外周血管疾病病史的患者在标准治疗即阿司匹林、氯吡格雷或阿司匹林联合氯吡格雷（58%DAPT）基础上接受沃拉帕沙 2.5mg，1 次 / 日或安慰剂。中位数 30 个月结果显示，沃拉帕沙显著降低心肌梗死发生率从而使主要终点事件率（心血管原因死亡、心肌梗死或卒中）下降。但是沃拉帕沙组 GUSTO 研究（Global Utilisation of Strategies To open Occluded arteries）定义的中度或重度出血增加，颅内出血增加 2 倍，因而抵消了其抑制缺血事件的效果。

第 3 节　β- 受体阻滞剂

1. 早期静脉应用 β- 受体阻滞剂

溶栓治疗的患者早期静脉应用 β- 受体阻滞剂降低急性恶性室性心律失常的发生率，然而，没有明确的证据表明其有长期的临床获益。

在 PPCI 的患者，METOCARD-CNIC 研究（Effect of Metoprolol in Cardioprotection During an Acute Myocardial Infarction）（270 例）显示，对没有心力衰竭征象并且收缩压 > 120mmHg 的前壁 STEMI 患者在确诊时极早期静脉使用美托洛尔（15mg），与对照组相比，其 5 ～ 7 天时磁共振测量的梗死面积减小（25.6g 与 32.0g；*P* = 0.012）、6 个月时磁共振测量的左心室射血分数提高（48.7% *vs.* 45.0%；*P*=0.018）提高。研究中所有无禁忌的患者 24 小时内接受了口服美托洛尔。2 年的 MACE（死亡、因心力衰竭再住院、再次心肌梗死和恶性室性心律失常的复合终点）发病率在静脉美托洛尔组和对照组分别为 10.8% *vs.* 18.3%（*P*=0.065）。美托洛尔治疗与微循环栓塞的发生率和程度降低显著相关。EARLY-BAMI 研究（Early Intravenous Beta-Blockers in Patients With ST–Segment Elevation Myocardial Infarction Before Primary Percutaneous Coronary Intervention）将 683 例发病 12 小时内的 STEMI 患者随机分为静脉美托洛尔组（在入组时给予 5mg，PCI 之前再次给予 5mg）或安慰剂组，所有无禁忌证的患者 12 小时内接受口服美托洛尔治疗。结果显示，早期静脉应用美托洛尔组没有减少磁共振测定的梗死面积 [研究的主要终点仅在 342 例（55%）患者中获得] 或降低心肌生物标志物释放水平。早期静脉应用美托洛尔组减少恶性室性心律失常发生率（3.6% vs. 6.9%，P=0.050）。30 天随访结果显示，早期静脉应用美托洛尔组患者没有出现血流动力学不稳定、房室传导阻滞或 MACE。有关 PPCI 研究的事后分析结果显示，早期静脉应用 β - 受体阻滞剂可能与临床获益相关，但是不能排除即使在校正基线特征的不平衡之后还是存在选择偏倚。基于现有的证据，对于血流动力学稳定的 PPCI 的患者，应当考虑症状发生早期静脉应用并随后口服 β - 受体阻滞剂。

2. 中期和长期的 β - 受体阻滞剂

尽管大部分的证据来自再灌注时代以前研究，STEMI 后长期口服 β - 受体阻滞剂的获益已十分明确（表 7–3）。最近的一项多中心注册登记研究连续入选 7057 例急性心肌梗死患者，平均随访 2.1 年的结果显示，β - 受体阻滞剂在降低死亡率方面的获益与出院时处方 β - 受体阻滞剂相关，不过没有发现剂量与结果相关。有研究利用注册数据分析了 19 843 例 ACS 或接受 PCI 的患者使用新型 β - 受体阻滞剂对心血管事件的影响。平均随访 3.7 年的结果显示，β - 受体阻滞剂的应用与死亡率显著减少相关（校正的 HR=0.90，95%CI：0.84 ～ 0.96）。β - 受体阻滞剂和结果之间的关联在有或没有近期心肌梗死的患者之间差异显著（死亡 HR=0.85 vs. 1.02；P= 0.007）。不过，一项纳入 6758 例既往心肌梗死患者的回顾追踪倾向匹配研究并没有显示 β - 受体阻滞剂可以降低心血管事件或死亡率。基于目前的证据，如心力衰竭指南中详细讨论的那样，应当考虑在所有 STEMI 患者中常规应用 β - 受体阻滞剂。没有禁忌证（如急性心力衰竭、血流动力学不稳定或高度房室传导阻滞）的左心室收缩功能降低（LVEF ≤ 40%）的患者建议应用 β - 受体阻滞剂，应给予证明有效的药物和剂量。迄今 β - 受体阻滞剂维持用药时间的问题还没有研究回答，所以这方面还不能给出建

表 7-3　急性期、亚急性期和慢性期常规治疗药物：β-受体阻滞剂、血管紧张素转换酶抑制剂、血管紧张素Ⅱ受体阻滞剂、盐皮质激素受体拮抗剂和降脂治疗

建议	建议类别	证据水平
β-受体阻滞剂		
除非有禁忌证，心力衰竭和（或）LVEF ≤ 40% 的患者应该口服 β-受体阻滞剂	I	A
对没有禁忌证、急性心力衰竭并且收缩压 > 120mmHg 准备行直接 PCI 的患者，应该考虑静脉途径使用 β-受体阻滞剂	Ⅱa	A
没有禁忌证的患者，住院期间及出院后应该常规口服 β-受体阻滞剂	Ⅱa	B
低血压、急性心力衰竭、房室传导阻滞或严重心动过缓的患者，应避免静脉使用 β-受体阻滞剂	Ⅲ	B
降脂治疗		
除非有禁忌证，建议尽早启动高强度他汀治疗[a]并长期维持	I	A
建议将 LDL-C 降至 < 1.8mmol/L（70mg/dl）；如果基线 LDL-C 在 1.8～3.5mmol/L（70～135mg/dl）之间则至少降低 50%	I	B
对所有 STEMI 患者就诊后尽早行血脂谱检查	I	C
高危患者尽管使用最大耐受剂量他汀治疗 LDL-C 水平仍 ≥ 1.8mmol/L（70mg/dl）时，应该考虑进一步降 LDL-C 治疗	Ⅱa	A
ACEI/ARB		
合并心力衰竭、左室收缩功能不全、糖尿病或前壁心肌梗死的 STEMI 患者，建议在 24 小时内启动 ACEI 治疗	I	A
在合并心力衰竭和（或）左心室收缩功能不全患者，可以使用 ARB（优选缬沙坦）替代 ACEI，尤其是不能耐受 ACEI 时	I	B
只要没有禁忌证，所有患者都应使用 ACEI	Ⅱa	A
盐皮质激素受体拮抗剂		
若无肾衰竭或高钾血症，对合并糖尿病或者已经使用 ACEI 和 β-受体阻滞剂的情况下 LVEF 仍 ≤ 40% 和心力衰竭的患者，建议使用盐皮质激素受体拮抗剂	I	B

注：[a] 定义为阿托伐他汀 40～80mg 或瑞舒伐他汀 20～40mg。

议。关于未早期使用静脉 β - 受体阻滞剂的患者开始口服 β - 受体阻滞剂的时机问题，一项纳入 5259 例患者的回顾性注册分析显示，早期（＜ 24 小时）口服 β - 受体阻滞剂与延迟给药相比有生存获益。因此，血流动力学稳定的患者应当考虑在第一个 24 小时之内开始口服 β - 受体阻滞剂。

第 4 节　降脂治疗

他汀类药物用于二级预防的获益已相当明确。研究也证实 ACS 患者早期强化他汀治疗有益。一项荟萃分析对比了较高强度强化和较低强度强化他汀降低 LDL-C 的效果。结果显示，较高强度强化他汀类治疗明显降低心血管死亡、非致死性心肌梗死、缺血性卒中和冠状动脉血运重建的风险。LDL-C 每降低 1mmol/L 所达成的风险降低程度与他汀和安慰剂比较的研究中的降低程度相当。因此，建议所有急性心肌梗死患者服用他汀类药物，而不考虑就诊时胆固醇水平。降脂治疗应尽早开始，这样可以增加患者出院后的依从性。高强度他汀治疗与早期和持续临床获益相关，所以应尽可能给予高强度他汀的治疗。除非有不能耐受高强度他汀类治疗的病史或有其他用药安全性的问题，对于就诊时已接受低或中等强度他汀治疗的患者应当增加他汀类药物治疗的强度。治疗目标是 LDL-C ＜ 1.8mmol/ L（＜ 70mg/dl），如果基线 LDL-C 水平为 1.8 ～ 3.5mmol/ L，则至少降低 50%。他汀类药物不良反应风险增加的患者应当考虑较低强度的他汀类治疗（如老年、肝损伤或肾损伤、曾发生过不良反应或与合并用药存在潜在的相互作用）。心肌梗死后血脂谱呈时相性变化，第一个 24 小时内总胆固醇、LDL-C 和 HDL-C 轻微降低，而甘油三酯增加。STEMI 患者就诊后应尽可能早地获得血脂谱。可以是非空腹的，因为总胆固醇和 HDL-C 昼夜变化较小，而 LDL-C 的变化范围在 10% 以内。ACS 患者 4 ～ 6 周后应重新评估血脂谱，以确定是否已经达到目标水平并评价用药安全性问题，然后可以根据病情相应地调整降脂治疗。高剂量阿托伐他汀和辛伐他汀用药的研究结果支持高强度他汀类药物治疗。

不能耐受任何剂量他汀类药物的患者，应当考虑使用应用依折麦布。IMPROVE-IT 研究（Improved . Reduction of Outcomes: Vytorin Efficacy International Trial）涉及了 18 144 例有近期 ACS（29% 为 STEMI）的患者，随机分组为依折麦布 10mg 联合辛伐他汀 40mg 组或单独辛伐他汀 40mg 组（如果 LDL-C ＞ 79mg/dl 或 2.04mmol/L，辛伐他汀剂量则逐渐滴定至 80mg）。7 年随访结果显示，与他汀类药物单用相比，联合药物治疗组心血管死亡、心肌梗死、因不稳定型心绞痛住院、冠状动脉血运重建或卒中的复合主要终点事件发生率明显降低（32.7% *vs.* 34.7%，*HR*=0.94，95%*CI*：0.89 ～ 0.99）。

最近的 Ⅰ ～ Ⅲ 期临床试验数据表明，前蛋白转化酶枯草溶菌素 9（proprotein convertase subtilisin/kexin type 9， PCSK9）抑制剂不论是单独使用还是联合他汀治疗能降低 LDL-C 最高达 60%。PCSK9 抑制剂还有降低甘油三酯和升高 HDL-C 的有益效果。超过 10 000 例患者的临床研究的荟萃分析显示，PCSK9 抑制剂显著降低死亡率（*HR*=0.45，95%*CI*：0.23 ～ 0.86）。不过，该研究中的终点事件较少。FOURIER（Cardiovascular Outcomes Research with PCSK9 Inhibition in Subjects with Elevated Risk）研究纳入了 27 564 例动脉粥样硬化性心血管疾病患者，这些患者有其他危险因素、LDL-C ≥ 70mg/dl（1.8mmol/L）并且已接收中等或高强度的他汀类药物治疗。与安慰剂组相比，注射依伏库单抗（evolocumab）可使心血管死亡、心肌梗死、卒中、因不稳定型心绞痛住院或冠状血管重建的主要复合终点事件相对减少 15%、绝对降低 1.5%。两组之间全因死亡或心血管死亡发生率及不良事件发生率没有差异。鉴于 2 年使用效果中等并且没有降低死亡率，依伏库单抗应仅限于一些高风险的患者使用。

基于相对有限的证据，高风险 STEMI 患者使用最大耐受剂量他汀仍不能达到治疗目标时应当考虑加用非他汀类药物治疗。

第 5 节 硝酸酯类

一项随机对照试验显示，STEMI 患者常规应用硝酸酯类与安慰剂相比没有获益，因此不建议使用。如果没有低血压、右心室梗死或在 48 小时内使用 5 型磷酸二酯酶抑制剂，合并高血压或心力衰竭的患者在急性期静脉应用硝酸盐可能有用。急性期之后，硝酸盐对于控制残余心绞痛症状有帮助。

第 6 节 钙拮抗药

一项涉及 17 项针对 STEMI 患者早期应用钙拮抗药的临床试验的荟萃分析显示，钙拮抗药不能降低死亡或再梗死，硝苯地平还有增加死亡率的趋势。因此，在急性期不建议常规应用钙拮抗药。一项随机对照试验将 1775 例未接受 β - 受体阻滞剂的心肌梗死慢性期患者分为维拉帕米组或安慰剂组，结果发现维拉帕米组死亡和再梗死的危险性降低。因此，对于有 β - 受体阻滞剂禁忌证尤其是合并阻塞性气道疾病的患者，在没有心力衰竭或左室功能受损的情况下可以选择钙拮抗药。此外，STEMI之后常规使用二氢吡啶类药物没有获益。因此，只有存在其他明确适应证（如高血压或残余心绞痛）时才能使用此类药物。

第 7 节 血管紧张素转换酶抑制剂和血管紧张素 II 受体阻滞剂

建议左心室功能受损（LVEF ≤ 40%）或早期发生心力衰竭的患者使用 ACEI。STEMI 患者早期应用 ACEI 的荟萃分析显示，ACEI 治疗安全、耐受性良好，并且能小幅度降低 30 天死亡率（有统计学意义），大部分在第一周见到获益。ACEI

不仅用于左心室收缩功能不全、心力衰竭、高血压或糖尿病患者，所有 STEMI 患者都应考虑使用 ACEI。不耐受 ACEI 的患者应给予血管紧张素 II 受体阻滞剂（angiotensin II receptor blocker，ARB）。VALIANT 研究显示（VALsartan In Acute myocardial iNfarcTion），对于 STEMI 患者缬沙坦效果不劣于卡托普利。

第 8 节　盐皮质激素和醛固酮受体拮抗剂

建议 STEMI 后左心室功能不全（LVEF ≤ 40%）和心力衰竭的患者应用盐皮质激素受体拮抗剂（mineralocorticoid receptor antagonist，MRA）。依普利酮是一种选择性醛固酮受体拮抗剂，能够降低这类患者的发病率和死亡率。EPHESUS 研究（Eplerenone Post-AMI Heart failure Efficacy and SUrvival Study）纳入 6642 例心肌梗死后左室功能不全（LVEF ≤ 40%）并有心力衰竭症状和（或）糖尿病的患者，在心肌梗死后 3 ～ 14 天随机给予依普利酮或安慰剂治疗。平均随访 16 个月的结果显示，依普利酮使总死亡率相对降低 15%，死亡和因心血管事件住院的复合终点降低 13%。

最近的两项研究显示没有心力衰竭的 STEMI 患者早期使用 MRA 获益。REMINDER 研究（Double-Blind，Randomized，Placebo-Controlled Trial Evaluating The Safety And Efficacy Of Early Treatment With Eplerenone In Patients With Acute Myocardial Infarction）随机选取 1012 例无心力衰竭的急性 STEMI 患者在症状出现后 24 小时内应用依普利酮或安慰剂。10.5 个月后依普利酮组主要联合终点 [心血管死亡、再住院、因心力衰竭延长初次住院时间、持续室性心动过速或室颤、射血分数 ≤ 40%，或 B 型钠尿肽（B-type natriuretic peptide，BNP）/ N- 末端 B 型利钠肽（N-terminal pro B-type natriuretic peptide，NT-proBNP）水平升高] 发生率低于安慰剂组（18.2% *vs.* 29.4%，$P < 0.0001$），其差异主要由 BNP 水平差异导致。ALBATROSS 研究（Aldosterone Lethal effects Blockade in Acute myocardial infarction Treated with or without Reperfusion to improve Outcome and Survival at Six months follow-up）入选了 1603 例急性 STEMI 或高

风险 NSTEMI 患者，随机分为单次静脉推注坎利酸钾（potassium canrenoate）200mg 之后应用螺内酯（每日 25mg）组和安慰剂组。总体上，两组间 6 个月复合终点（死亡、心脏骤停复苏、严重室性心律失常、置入式除颤器适应证或者新发或恶化的心力衰竭）没有差异。针对 STEMI 亚组（1229 例）的探索性分析显示，治疗组的复合终点明显降低（*HR*=0.20；95%*CI*：0.06 ～ 0.70）。MRA 对 STEMI 患者的作用需进一步研究阐明。

肾功能降低 [男性肌酐浓度＞ 221mmol/L（2.5mg/dl），女性＞ 177mmol/L（2.0mg/dl）] 时应用 MRA 要谨慎，必须常规监测血钾浓度。

图 7-1 和图 7-2 展示 PPCI 或溶栓治疗时的常用药物处方（Ⅰ类和Ⅱa 类）。

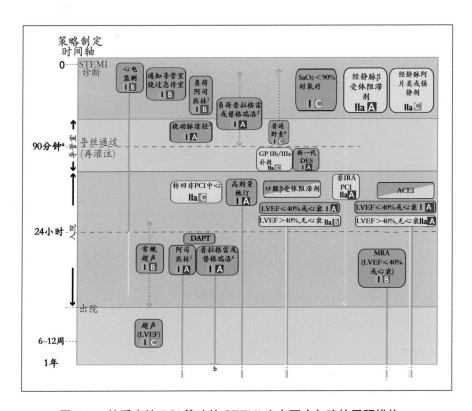

图 7-1　接受直接 PCI 策略的 STEMI 患者不应忽略的干预措施

注：ACEI：血管紧张素转换酶抑制剂；DAPT：双联抗血小板治疗；DES：药物涂层支架；IRA：梗死相关动脉；LVEF：左室射血分数；MRA：盐皮质激素受体拮抗剂；PCI：经皮冠状动脉介入治疗；STEMI：ST 段抬高型心肌梗死。

本图展示了最应遵守的干预措施（Ⅰ类绿色，Ⅱa 类黄色）和预期干预时间。实线代表周期性（每日）的干预措施。双箭头虚线表示某种措施可以实施的时间窗。

[1] 阿司匹林负荷量：150 ～ 300mg 嚼服或 75 ～ 250mg 静脉推注（适用于未服用阿司匹林维持量的患者）。

[2] 普拉格雷负荷量：60mg。替格瑞洛负荷量：180mg。如果普拉格雷或替格瑞洛无药或有禁忌证，则给予氯吡格雷负荷量 600mg。

[3] 如果介入医师不擅长桡动脉途径，则应选择股动脉途径。

[4] 可以用依诺肝素或比伐卢定替代普通肝素（Ⅱ a A 级）。

[5] 阿司匹林维持量：75 ～ 100mg 口服。

[6] 普拉格雷维持量：10mg qd。替格瑞洛维持量：90mg bid。如果普拉格雷或替格瑞洛无药或有禁忌证，则给予氯吡格雷维持量 75mg qd。

[a] 90 分钟代表到 PCI 再灌注治疗所需的最长时间间隔。对于首诊于 PCI 中心的患者，这一目标时间为 60min。

[b] 可耐受 DAPT 且无出血并发症的高缺血风险患者，可以考虑阿司匹林联合替格瑞洛 60mg bid 延长使用至 36 个月。

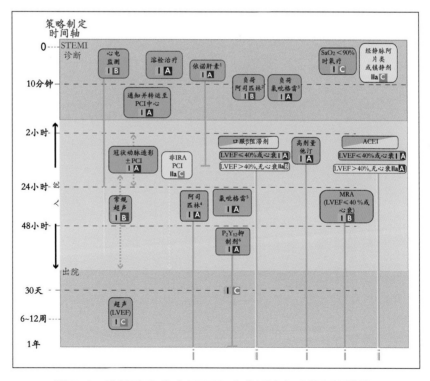

图 7-2　溶栓治疗成功 STEMI 患者不应忽略的干预措施

注：ACEI：血管紧张素转换酶抑制剂；IRA：梗死相关动脉；LVEF：左室射血分数；MRA：盐皮质激素受体拮抗剂；PCI 经皮冠状动脉介入治疗；STEMI：ST 段抬高型心肌梗死。

本图展示了最应遵守的干预措施（Ⅰ类绿色，Ⅱa类黄色）和预期干预时间。实线代表周期性（每日）的干预措施。双箭头虚线表示某种措施可以实施的时间窗。

^{1} 依诺肝素剂量：30mg 负荷量静脉推注后每 12 小时以 1mg/kg 剂量皮下注射给药（对于 ≥ 75 岁及肾功能不全患者的剂量调整见表 6-2）。

^{2} 阿司匹林负荷量：150 ～ 300mg 嚼服，或 75 ～ 250mg 静脉推注。

^{3} 氯吡格雷负荷量：300mg 口服（≥ 75 岁人群使用 75mg）。

^{4} 阿司匹林维持量：75 ～ 100mg 口服

^{5} 氯吡格雷维持量：75mg qd

^{6} 接受 PCI 治疗的患者可以考虑在溶栓 48 小时后换用普拉格雷或替格瑞洛。

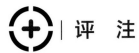

评 注

本章讨论了 STEMI 患者的生活方式干预和危险因素控制、抗栓药物治疗和非抗栓药物治疗 3 个方面的内容。

全面进行生活方式干预和危险因素控制对于改善 STEMI 患者的预后非常重要。但是在国内的临床实践中并没有引起重视，即使患者到门诊复查时，鲜有医师进行专门的指导。在控制危险因素中，首先应当强调控制体重。STEMI 患者往往重视药物治疗，却忽视了控制体重的重要性。实际上，如果能够良好地控制体重，患者的高血压、高脂血症和高糖血症则更容易控制。此外，要强调适当活动和心脏康复训练的重要性。

在早期治疗时就实施二级预防患者教育能够明显提供患者出院后的依从性。然而，国内在此方面重视不够。一方面是患者太多，医务人员无暇顾及，另一方面是缺乏相关专业的人员。因此，国内亟待加强这方面的工作，以提高患者治疗的长期效果。

DAPT 是 STEMI 患者（尤其是接受了 PCI 的患者）出院后的重要治疗。在我们编辑出版的《解读欧洲冠心病抗血小板治疗指南 . 2018》中有详细讨论，在此不再赘述。

非抗栓药物治疗包括应用 β - 受体阻滞剂、降脂治疗和应用硝酸酯类、钙拮抗药、血管紧张素转换酶抑制剂和血管紧张素 Ⅱ 受体阻滞剂、盐皮质激素和醛固酮受体拮抗剂，指南均有详述。然而，临床实践中经常看到对这些药物的应用没有采取个体化方案，并且动态进行调整，往往变成了"套餐"式的用药。新近的研究对于现代条件下长期常规应用 β - 受体阻滞剂的价值提出了挑战，显示这种做法并不能降低 STEMI 患者的长期死亡率。硝酸酯类经常是 STEMI 患者出院后长期常规用药。实际上，在已经获得完全血运重建的 STEMI 患者，没有必要长期应用。应用钙拮抗药时要考虑多数钙拮抗药对心脏功能的影响。对于严重心功能不全或需要合并用药的 STEMI 患者，应当首先选择血管紧张素转换酶抑制剂，而不是血管紧张素 Ⅱ 受体阻滞剂。但是国内不问青红皂白首先选择血管紧张素 Ⅱ 受体阻滞剂的情况并非少见。盐皮质激素和醛固酮受体拮抗剂应当应用于有适应证的患者。总之，临床医师应当根据患者的情况选择用药，并且动态调整，避免"one size fit all"。

第八章
ST 段抬高型心肌梗死的并发症

第 1 节　心肌功能紊乱

STEMI 急性期和亚急性期可能发生左室功能不全。取决于缺血时间的长短和再灌注是否完全，心功能不全可以是一过性（心肌顿抑）或持续性。早期心肌再灌注成功后心室功能通常得到改善（可能需要数周时间），但不是所有患者都有改善。

1. 左室功能不全

（1）**左室功能不全**　是 STEMI 最为常见的后果，也是死亡率的强预测因素。其原因是心肌损失或缺血性功能障碍（顿抑），当发生心律失常、瓣膜功能不全或机械并发症时加重。左室功能不全可以导致心力衰竭，也可以没有临床症状。其诊断依据临床表现和影像技术（超声心动图技术最为常用）。

（2）**左室室壁瘤**　不到 5% 的大面积透壁心肌梗死患者会发生负性重构形成左室室壁瘤。室壁瘤患者心力衰竭发生率高，应当根据有关指南进行治疗。外科室壁瘤切除似乎不获益。但是，大室壁瘤患者当心力衰竭不能控制、反复发生消融不能纠正的室性心律失常时可以考虑外科手术治疗。

（3）**左室血栓**　左室血栓是前壁心肌梗死常见的并发症（即使没有心尖部室壁瘤）。附壁血栓诊断一旦确立，应在超声心动图复查、权衡出血风险和抗血小板治疗的基础上进行不超过 6 个月的口服抗凝治疗。不过，目前还缺乏前瞻性研究评估最佳的抗凝方案和时间，以及合并使用抗血小板药物的策略，直接口服抗凝药治疗附壁血栓的临床经验也非常有限。其他临床情况联合使用抗凝药和抗血小板药的建议已有指南发表。

（4）继发性二尖瓣反流　左室重构造成侧壁和心尖乳头肌位移、瓣叶牵拉和瓣环扩张是导致继发性（功能性）二尖瓣反流的常见原因。继发性二尖瓣反流多数属于晚期并发症。不过，大面积心肌梗死尤其是累及左室后侧壁造成后内侧乳头肌明显功能不全时，也可能在亚急性期出现继发性二尖瓣反流。经胸超声心动图是初步诊断继发性二尖瓣反流的重要手段，有时还可能需要进行经食管超声心动图检查进一步明确二尖瓣反流的机制和程度。再灌注和强化药物治疗（包括利尿剂、动脉血管扩张剂）可以改善二尖瓣反流的程度。严重二尖瓣反流患者反复发生心力衰竭或血流动力学不稳定，并且对上述治疗无反应时，应进行紧急或急诊二尖瓣手术。对于这类患者，尽管总死亡率较高，但是二尖瓣置换改善生存和左心室功能的效果优于单纯药物治疗。

2.心肌梗死累及右室

心肌梗死累及右室最常见于下壁STEMI。右室心肌梗死可以根据aVR、V_1和（或）右室心前导联（V_3R和V_4R）ST段抬高≥1mm诊断。下壁STEMI患者应常规做右心室心前导联心电图。超声心动图常常用来确定右室心肌梗死，心脏磁共振评价右心室心肌梗死效果也较好。右心室心肌梗死的病程可以较为单纯，或者表现有典型三联征（低血压、肺野清晰和颈静脉压升高）。右心室心肌梗死也容易合并室性心律失常、房室传导阻滞、机械并发症、低心输出量和休克。右心室缺血的治疗包括：早期再灌注（尤其要注意开通右室支），可以迅速改善血流动力学；避免使用降低前负荷的药物（硝酸酯类和利尿剂）；纠正房室不同步（纠正房颤）和（或）房室阻滞，必要时予以房室顺序起搏。

第 2 节　心力衰竭

1. 临床表现

心力衰竭是 STEMI 最常见的并发症和最重要的预后因素之一。STEMI 急性期诊断心力衰竭依据典型的临床症状、查体和胸片，并根据 Killip 分级进行风险评估。与慢性心力衰竭不同，BNP 诊断心肌梗死后急性心力衰竭的临界值还不明确，因而其应用价值有限。查明 STEMI 时心力衰竭的机制非常重要，左心室收缩功能不全是最常见的原因，还要评价是否由于血流动力学或心律不稳定、机械并发症和瓣膜功能不全所致。因此，必需尽早对患者进行经胸超声心动图检查，评价心肌损伤的范围、左心室收缩和舒张功能、左心室收缩和舒张期容积、瓣膜功能，以及机械并发症情况。任何突发伴有血流动力学受损的临床情况恶化都应进行临床再评估，包括复查超声心动图，尤其注意是否有左心室功能不全、二尖瓣反流或机械并发症进行性加重。

（1）**肺淤血**　可表现为轻中度肺淤血（Killip 2 级）至明显肺水肿（Killip 3 级），经再灌注和药物治疗后较快恢复或者演变为慢性心力衰竭，需依照当前有关指南进行处理。

（2）**低血压**　定义为收缩压＜ 90mmHg。有多种原因可以导致低血压，包括左室或右室功能不全、低心输出量、心律紊乱、机械并发症、瓣膜功能不全、低血容量或药物过量。低血压可以没有症状，也可以导致意识模糊或晕厥。长时间低血压可以导致急性肾功能不全或其他系统并发症。因此，严重低血压应当尽快予以纠正。

（3）**低心输出量**　表现为持续低血压和外周灌注不良（包括肾功能不全和尿量减少）。孤立性低心输出量最常见于严重右室心肌梗死患者，也可见于左室功能不全、二尖瓣反流或机械并发症患者。Doppler 超声是早期明确低血压并发症原因的必要手段。

（4）**心源性休克**　定义为容量充足的情况下持续低血压（收缩压＜ 90mmHg）伴有灌注不良表现。心源性休克占所有 STEMI 患者的 6% ～ 10%，目前依然是 STEMI 的首位死因，其院内死亡率≥ 50%。心源性休克在就诊前并不常见，半数发生于最初 6 小时以内，75% 发生在最初 24 小时以内。其典型表现是低血压，低心输出量（如静息时心动过速、精神状态改变、少尿和肢端发凉）和肺淤血。血流动力学表现包括心指数 $< 2.2L/(min \cdot m^2)$、楔嵌压 $> 18mmHg$ 和尿量 $< 20ml/h$。当需要正性肌力药和（或）机械循环辅助才能维持收缩压 $> 90mmHg$ 时也认为存在心源性休克。

心源性休克通常见于左室大面积梗死或右室心肌梗死。心源性休克死亡率可能与初始左室收缩功能和二尖瓣反流程度相关，其他指标如血清乳酸和肌酐水平也可以预测死亡率。早期超声心动图发现右室功能不全（尤其是双心室功能不全）也是预后不良的重要预测因素。因此，心源性休克不见得必须进行有创血流动力学监测，但是必须立即进行经胸超声心动图检查评估 LVEF 和机械并发症。

2. 处理

心力衰竭患者应予以持续监测心律、血压和尿量。应当尽快进行体格检查、心电图、超声心动图和有创血流动力学监测（病情不能迅速稳定时）来明确心力衰竭的原因，并尽早予以纠正（表 8-1）。

（1）肺淤血的处理　肺淤血伴有 $SaO_2 < 90\%$ 或氧分压（PaO_2）$< 60mmHg$（8.0kPa）时需要进行氧疗并进行 SaO_2 监测。纠正低氧血症的目标是 SaO_2 达到 95%，必要时定期进行血气分析。初步药物治疗包括：静推袢利尿剂（根据病情变化和尿量间断静脉使用呋塞米 20 ~ 40mg），如果血压允许可以静脉使用硝酸酯类（注意避免低血压和血压下降过度）。在没有低血压、低血容量或肾功能不全时建议早期使用 β - 受体阻滞剂、ACEI（或 ARB）和 MRA。必须进行病因治疗。CAD 严重时应当早期进行血运重建。心律紊乱、瓣膜功能不全和高血压应当尽早予以纠正。高血压应迅速给予口服 ACEI（或 ARB）和静脉硝酸酯类药物，严重高血压病例可能需要静脉泵入硝普钠。持续心肌缺血应当早期进行血运重建。心房心室节律障碍、瓣膜功能不全或机械并发症应当酌情予以治疗。

肺淤血症状严重的患者可能需要静脉使用吗啡以减轻呼吸困难和焦虑。不过，吗啡可以引起恶心和呼吸抑制，不建议常规使用。无创正压通气（持续气道正压通气、双相气道正压通气）或高流量鼻导管吸氧治疗肺水肿有效，对于呼吸窘迫（呼吸频率＞ 25 次 / 分、SaO_2 ＜ 90%）的患者应尽快予以使用。对于不能达到足够氧合、呼吸做功过度或明确呼吸衰竭导致高碳酸血症的患者可予以气管插管和通气支持。利尿剂抵抗（尤其是低钠血症）的患者可以考虑进行超滤减少容量负荷。

表 8-1　ST 段抬高型心肌梗死后左室功能不全和急性心力衰竭的处理

建议	建议类别	证据水平
建议 LVEF ≤ 40% 和（或）心力衰竭患者在血流动力学稳定后尽早使用 ACEI（若不能耐受则使用 ARB），以减少住院和死亡风险	I	A
建议 LVEF ≤ 40% 和（或）心力衰竭患者稳定后使用 β - 受体阻滞剂，以减少死亡、再发心肌梗死及因心力衰竭再住院风险	I	A
若无严重肾功能不全和高钾血症，建议心力衰竭并且 LVEF ≤ 40% 的患者使用盐皮质激素受体拮抗剂，以减少心血管再住院和死亡风险	I	B
建议因容量负荷过重引起症状 / 体征的急性心力衰竭患者使用袢利尿剂以改善症状	I	C
有心力衰竭症状且收缩压＞ 90mmHg 的患者建议使用硝酸酯类以改善症状，减少淤血	I	C
SaO_2 ＜ 90% 的肺水肿患者建议氧疗，维持氧饱和度＞ 95%	I	C
因呼吸衰竭导致低氧血症、高碳酸血症或酸中毒患者，若不能耐受无创通气治疗则建议行气管插管	I	C
呼吸窘迫（呼吸频率＞ 25 次 / 分，SaO_2 ＜ 90%）患者若无低血压应该考虑行无创正压通气（持续气道正压、双相气道正压）	II a	B
合并心力衰竭和收缩压升高时，应该考虑静脉使用硝酸酯或硝普钠以控制血压、改善症状	II a	C
肺水肿和严重呼吸困难患者可以考虑使用阿片类药物以缓解呼吸困难和焦虑。应该监测患者呼吸情况	II b	B
严重心力衰竭合并低血压经标准药物治疗无效的患者，可以考虑使用正性肌力药	II b	C

对于血压尚能维持（收缩压＞90mmHg）但心输出量严重下降影响重要脏器灌注，经标准治疗无改善的心力衰竭患者，可以考虑使用多巴酚丁胺或左西孟旦。不过，目前心源性休克使用左西孟旦的临床经验有限。有关急性心力衰竭临床处理的详细内容可以查阅2016年版ESC《急性和慢性心力衰竭诊断与治疗指南》。

（2）**低血压的处理**　对于血压低而组织灌注正常的患者，如果没有淤血、容量负荷过重（下腔静脉塌陷）和并发症（机械并发症或严重二尖瓣反流），应当在监测中心静脉压条件下适当补充容量。心动过缓或心动过速应当予以纠正或控制。右室心肌梗死患者应当避免容量负荷过重，因其可能导致血流动力学恶化。如果存在持续性低血压，可以考虑使用正性肌力药物（优选多巴酚丁胺）。

（3）**心源性休克的处理**　治疗心源性休克首先是明确病因并纠正可逆性因素，如血容量不足、药物导致的低血压或心律失常。特殊因素如机械并发症、心脏压塞等导致的心源性休克应予以针对性治疗（表8-2）。

1）STEMI合并心源性休克患者预计到PCI再灌注时间超过120min时，应当立即予以溶栓治疗并转运至PCI中心。到达PCI中心后不论ST段是否回落和溶栓后时间长短，都应当立即进行急诊冠状动脉造影。

2）STEMI合并心源性休克应尽可能实施PPCI进行再灌注，多支病变时予以完全血运重建。对于发生心源性休克风险高的患者，在其出现血流动力学不稳定之前尽早转运至区域性中心治疗可能有益。心源性休克患者的抗心律失常治疗同其他STEMI患者的治疗没有区别。右室心肌梗死相关的低心输出量心源性休克治疗的特殊性问题见本章第1节和第2节。

3）建议进行动脉系统有创血压监测。可以采用肺动脉压监测，以便准确调节充盈压、评估心输出量或不明原因休克。首先要除外低血容量并予以补液纠正。药物治疗的目的是通过提高心输出量和血压改善器官灌注。能够保障有适当的组织灌注时，建议予以利尿治疗。通常需要静脉使用正性肌力药和血管升压药，以维持收缩压＞90mmHg并提高心输出量、改善重要器官灌注。低心输出量占主要原因的患者初步治疗可使用多巴酚丁胺。对于心源性休克合并严重低血压的患者，去甲肾上腺素可能较多巴胺更加安全有效。左西孟旦的正性肌力作用不依赖于β肾上腺能激动，可以作为备选使用（尤其是对于长期使用 β - 受体阻滞剂的患者）。STEMI 不建议使用磷酸二酯酶Ⅲ抑制剂。

表 8-2　ST 段抬高型心肌梗死后心源性休克的处理

建议	分类	水平
心源性休克患者若冠脉解剖适宜，建议即刻实施 PCI。如果冠脉解剖不适宜 PCI 或 PCI 失败，则建议行急诊 CABG	Ⅰ	B
建议经动脉途径行有创血压监测	Ⅰ	C
建议行即刻行多普勒超声心电图检查，以评估心室和瓣膜功能，容量负荷状态以及检测有无机械并发症	Ⅰ	C
若出现机械并发症，建议由心脏病团队讨论后尽快处理	Ⅰ	C
根据患者血气结果决定是否给予氧疗或机械辅助通气	Ⅰ	C
心源性休克患者若无法在 STEMI 诊断后 120min 内实施直接 PCI，在排除机械并发症后应该考虑进行溶栓治疗	Ⅱa	C
心源性休克患者应该考虑在当次手术中行完全血运重建	Ⅱa	C
因机械并发症出现血流动力学不稳定或心源性休克的患者，应该考虑使用 IABP	Ⅱa	C
可以考虑行肺动脉导管血流动力学监测以明确诊断并指导治疗	Ⅱb	B
难治性心力衰竭患者对以利尿剂为基础的治疗无反应时，可以考虑行血液超滤治疗	Ⅱb	B
为稳定血流动力学可以考虑使用正性肌力药或血管收缩药	Ⅱb	C
难治性休克患者可以考虑短期使用机械辅助装置	Ⅱb	C
不建议常规使用 IABP	Ⅲ	B

4）不建议常规应用 IABP 反搏。IABP 反搏对于没有机械并发症的 STEMI 心源性休克患者没有改善预后的作用，也不能限制大面积前壁心肌梗死患者的梗死面积，因而不建议常规应用。不过，有些患者如严重二尖瓣关闭不全或室间隔破裂，可以考虑使用 IABP 反搏进行血流动力学支持。一项小规模探索性试验显示，急性心肌梗死合并心源性休克患者使用 Impella CP 经皮循环辅助装置与 IABP 相比没

有获益。

5）对于标准治疗（正性肌力药、液体调整和 IABP）没有反应的患者，目前，使用机械左室辅助装置包括短期经皮机械循环辅助装置即心内轴流泵和动脉静脉体外膜氧合获益的证据有限。因此，短期机械循环辅助装置可以作为某些患者心肌功能恢复、心脏移植或长期左室辅助治疗之前的桥接措施，以便稳定病情或保证器官灌注或氧合。

第 3 节　急性期心律失常和传导异常的处理

STEMI 早期数小时内经常发生心律失常和传导障碍，并且是影响预后的主要因素。尽管对 STEMI 急性期心律失常的认识和基础与高级生命支持都有了提高，其院前阶段心源性猝死的发生率仍然较高，主要原因是快速性室性心律失常（室速）和室颤。早期再灌注治疗降低室性心律失常和心血管死亡风险。STEMI 发生致命性心律失常需要进行快速完全地紧急血运重建。抗心律失常药物对 STEMI 患者效果的证据有限，有研究显示其对早期死亡率存在负面影响。建议谨慎使用抗心律失常药物或者采用其他方法，包括电复律、对血流动力学影响小或没有影响的心律失常采取密切观察策略，或者对某些患者进行心脏起搏或导管消融。建议纠正电解质失衡，早期应用 β-受体阻滞剂、ACEI（或 ARB）和他汀。

1. 室上性心动过速

最常见的室上性心动过速为房颤，最高可占 STEMI 患者的 21%。房颤可能是既往存在首次发现，也可能是首次发作。房颤患者合并症较多，并发症风险也较高。除了需要抗凝治疗外，多数患者对房颤的耐受性较好不需要特殊治疗。几乎没有资料提示房颤血流动力学不稳定时进行心率控制优于节律控制，应当迅速进行电复律。但是，电复律成功后的早期复发率较高。房颤的处理见表 8-3。急性期节律控制药物仅限于使用胺碘酮，心率控制可以使用 β - 受体阻滞剂。大面积心肌梗死或严重左室功能不全的患者静脉应用地高辛（单用或与静脉胺碘酮合用）更为安全有效。静脉联合使用地高辛和胺碘酮可能导致地高辛血浓度升高，因此必须密切监测地高辛毒性。有些研究（不是所有）显示 β - 受体阻滞剂、ACEI（或 ARB）和早期他汀治疗可以减少新发房颤。房颤合并血栓栓塞危险因素的患者应当长期口服抗凝治疗。STEMI 合并房颤患者的短期和长期预后较窦性心律患者差。合并房颤患者的再梗死、卒中、心力衰竭和心源性猝死概率较高。研究显示，即便是 STEMI 期间自行终止的房颤，其与长期随访期间卒中率增加也存在相关性。

表 8-3　房颤的处理

建议	建议类别	证据水平
房颤发作时心率控制		
若没有急性心力衰竭和低血压，建议必要时静脉使用 β - 受体阻滞剂	I	C
若存在急性心力衰竭但无低血压时，建议必要时静脉使用胺碘酮	I	C
若存在急性心力衰竭和低血压，建议必要时静脉使用洋地黄制剂	II a	B
心律转复		
房颤患者合并持续心肌缺血、严重血流动力学障碍或心力衰竭，通过药物治疗仍不能有效地控制心率时，建议立即进行电转复	I	C
新发房颤病情不稳定的患者，建议使用静脉胺碘酮以提高电转复成功率，并减少早期复发风险	I	C
STEMI 急性期新发房颤的患者，应该考虑根据 CHA2DS2-VASc 评分行长期口服抗凝，并同时顾及抗栓药物合并用药	II a	C
地高辛对转复新发房颤无效，也不建议其用于节律控制	III	A
钙拮抗药和 β - 受体阻滞剂包括索他洛尔对转复新发房颤无效	III	B
不建议预防性使用抗心律失常药物预防房颤发作	III	B

注：CHA2DS2-VASc：心力衰竭、高血压、≥ 75 岁（2 分）、糖尿病、卒中（2 分）- 血管疾病、65 ~ 74 岁及性别（女性）；STEMI：ST 段抬高型心肌梗死。

2. 室性心律失常

近几十年来，STEMI 患者室速和室颤的发生率有所下降，主要归因于再灌注治疗和 β - 受体阻滞剂的使用。不过，仍有 6% ～ 8% 的患者发生影响血流动力学的室速或室颤。典型的心律失常表现为不稳定、多型性和频率相对较快的室速，容易演变为室颤。心肌缺血经常诱发这类心律失常，因而紧急血运重建至关重要。如果没有禁忌证，建议使用 β - 受体阻滞剂。必要时可以反复进行电复律或电除颤。控制效果不佳时应当静脉使用胺碘酮。胺碘酮禁忌时可以静脉应用利多卡因，但是目前还缺乏研究比较 STEMI 应用胺碘酮和利多卡因的优劣性。STEMI 前 48 小时内室速（室颤）对预后影响的结论还不一致，有研究显示早期室速（室颤）增加 30 天死亡率，但是不增加长期心律失常风险。

冠状动脉血流恢复时发生的室速或室颤（再灌注心律失常），其对于长期预后而言是良性的，因而不必进行药物抗心律失常治疗。室性期前收缩在急性期第一天非常多见，通常表现为复杂心律失常（多形室性期前收缩、短阵室速或 R-on-T 现象）。其预测室颤的价值不确定，也不需要特殊治疗。STEMI 早期（通常指发病 48 小时以内）时间窗以外的非缺血性持续性室速或室颤提示患者预后差，建议依据相关指南评估埋藏式心律转复除颤器置入作为心源性猝死二级预防的指征。心肌梗死 40 天内没有发生室速（室颤）时，通常不建议置入埋藏式心律转复除颤器进行心源性猝死的一级预防。对于既往因 LVEF 受损考虑有埋藏式心律转复除颤器一级预防指征的心肌梗死后早期患者，应当在血管重建后 6 ～ 12 周重新评估埋藏式心律转复除颤器置入指征。

有些患者即便接受了完全血运重建和抗心律失常药物治疗，仍然会发生电风暴和（或）持续性室速，可以采用超速起搏控制病情。不过，终止超速起搏后室速（室颤）复发率较高，此时导管消融可能是唯一的治疗手段，射频消融术成功可以终止室速（室颤）复发（表 8-4、表 8-5）。

表 8-4　急性期室性心律失常和传导阻滞的处理

建议	建议类别	证据水平
若没有禁忌证，对于多形性室速和（或）室颤患者建议静脉使用 β - 受体阻滞剂	I	B
再发室速和（或）室颤患者，建议迅速进行完全血运重建以纠正潜在的心肌缺血	I	C
建议静脉使用胺碘酮治疗再发多形性室速	I	C
建议对合并室速和（或）室颤患者纠正电解质紊乱（尤其是低钾血症和低镁血症）	I	C
窦性心动过缓合并血流动力学不稳定，或者高度房室传导阻滞不伴稳定性逸博心律时：		
建议静脉注射正性变时药物：肾上腺素、血管加压素和（或）阿托品	I	C
正性变时药物无效时，建议进行临时起搏	I	C
若患者尚未接受再灌注治疗，建议实施旨在血运重建的紧急冠状动脉造影	I	C
反复进行电转复仍有室速发作并伴有血流动力学不稳定的患者，应该考虑静脉使用胺碘酮	II a	C
反复电转复无法控制室速时，应该考虑经静脉导管起搏终止和（或）超速抑制起搏	II a	C
经完全血运重建和优化药物治疗后仍反复发作室速、室颤或心电风暴的患者，应该考虑行射频导管消融术，之后行 ICD 置入	II a	C
反复电转复室速仍然发作合并血流动力学障碍，在 β - 受体阻滞剂、胺碘酮和超速抑制起搏无效时，可以考虑使用利多卡因	II b	C
不建议预防性使用抗心律失常药物，并且可能有害	III	B
不建议使用抗心律失常药物治疗无症状或血流动力学稳定的室性心律失常	III	C

表 8-5　室性心律失常的长期管理和猝死风险评估

建议	建议类别	证据水平
已经优化药物治疗＞3个月并且心肌梗死后≥6周，仍然有症状性心力衰竭（NYHA Ⅱ～Ⅲ级）并且 LVEF≤35% 的患者，如果预期寿命≥1年且机体功能状态良好，建议置入 ICD 以减少猝死风险	Ⅰ	A
某些心肌梗死后＜40天的患者，包括非完全血运重建，存在基础左心功能不全，STEMI 发作48小时后发作心律失常、多形性室速或室颤，可以考虑置入 ICD 或短期使用可穿戴式心脏转复除颤器	Ⅱb	C

3. 窦性心动过缓和房室传导阻滞

窦性心动过缓在 STEMI 最初数小时内常见，有些病例可能是使用阿片类药物所致，通常不需要处理。STEMI 窦性心动过缓伴有严重低血压时应当静脉使用阿托品处理。二度Ⅰ型房室传导阻滞（莫氏Ⅰ型或文氏型）常见于下壁心肌梗死，罕见对血流动力学产生不良影响。如果影响了血流动力学，首先使用阿托品，无效时予以起搏治疗。应当慎用减慢房室传导的药物（如 β-受体阻滞剂、地高辛、维拉帕米或胺碘酮）。二度Ⅱ型房室传导阻滞（莫氏Ⅱ型）和完全性房室传导阻滞是起搏的指征。完全性房室传导阻滞、右室心肌梗死和血流动力学受损的患者应当考虑予以房室顺序起搏。没有进行再灌注治疗（如就诊延迟）的房室传导阻滞患者，应考虑予以血运重建。

下壁心肌梗死相关的房室传导阻滞多发生于希氏束以上部位，多在再灌注治疗后自行恢复。前壁心肌梗死相关的房室传导阻滞多发生在希氏束以下部位，由于大面积心肌坏死导致其死亡率较高。新发的束支阻滞或分支阻滞通常提示大面积前壁心肌梗死。高度房室传导阻滞伴有低逸搏心律、双分支或三分支阻滞时应考虑经静脉置入起搏电极。起搏的指征详见 ESC《心脏起搏与再同步化治疗指南》。

第 4 节　机械性并发症

机械并发症发生于 STEMI 后最初几天，在 PPCI 时代已明显减少。机械并发症威胁生命，需要迅速检查与处理。突发低血压、再发胸痛、新发提示二尖瓣反流或室间隔破裂的心脏杂音、肺淤血或颈静脉充盈时应怀疑出现机械并发症。怀疑机械并发症时应立即进行超声心动图检查。

1. 游离壁破裂

透壁心肌梗死后第一周有＜ 1% 的患者可能发生左室游离壁破裂，表现为突发胸痛和（或）心血管崩溃、伴或不伴有电机械分离。老年、未进行再灌注或者溶栓时间晚与心脏破裂发生率增加相关。心包积血和心脏压塞导致突发重度休克通常迅速死亡，超声心动图可以确诊。由于心脏破裂在三层心肌中呈现匍行性特征，有时血栓形成部分覆盖破裂部位和心包的限制作用有可能为心包穿刺、稳定血流动力学和随后的即刻外科手术争取到时间。建议采用心包补片（或其他材料）进行心室修补。取决于患者的状况和破裂的大小与形态，游离壁破裂的死亡率在 20% ～ 75%。病情允许的患者进行心脏磁共振检查有助于限制性心脏破裂的诊断并了解其解剖特点，从而指导外科手术干预。

2. 室间隔破裂

亚急性期发生室间隔破裂通常表现为临床情况迅速恶化，发生急性心力衰竭或心源性休克并伴有响亮的收缩期杂音。室间隔破裂可发生于 24 小时至数天，前壁和后侧壁心肌梗死发生室间隔破裂的概率相当。超声心动图和多普勒可以确诊室间隔破裂并与急性二尖瓣反流鉴别，还可以确定破裂的大小并定量左向右分流量。Swan-Ganz 导管可以更精确测定左向右分流量。左向右分流可导致新发急性右心衰竭。在准备冠状动脉造影和外科手术期间 IABP 支持可能有助于稳定患者的病情。低血压患者应当谨慎静脉使用利尿剂和血管扩张剂。室间隔破裂可能需要进行紧急外科修复，但是最佳手术时机目前还没有共识。早期手术的死亡率（文献报道为 20% ~ 40%）和再发心室破裂率高。延迟手术时瘢痕组织有利于室间隔修复，但是等待手术期间有室间隔破裂扩大和死亡的风险。因此，对于经积极治疗短期内没有反应的严重心力衰竭患者应早期进行手术修复。经积极纠正心力衰竭治疗反应良好的患者，可以考虑延期进行择期手术修复。采用设计恰当的器械进行经皮室间隔封堵术，有望成为外科手术之外可供选择的一项治疗措施。

3. 乳头肌断裂

急性心肌梗死后 2 ~ 7 天可能发生乳头肌或腱索断裂，从而导致急性二尖瓣反流。乳头肌断裂可以是完全断裂或是 1 个以上乳头肌断裂。由于后内侧乳头肌仅有一支动脉供血，其发生断裂的概率是其他乳头肌的 6 ~ 12 倍。 乳头肌断裂通常表现为血流动力学突然恶化伴有急性呼吸困难、肺水肿和（或）心源性休克。收缩期杂音经常被忽视。急诊超声心动图检查具有诊断意义。即刻治疗原则是降低后负荷来减轻反流和肺淤血。静脉应用利尿剂、血管扩张剂或正性肌力药以及 IABP 有助于稳定病情，为准备冠状动脉造影和手术争取时间。急诊手术是一个治疗选项，不过手术死亡率较高（20% ~ 25%）。手术时通常需要瓣膜置换，然而技术熟练的术者成功修复乳头肌结构的报道逐渐增多，可能是更好的选项。

第 5 节　心包炎

STEMI 心包并发症主要有 3 种：早期心肌梗死心包炎、后期心肌梗死心包炎（Dressler 综合征）和心包积液。

1. 早期心肌梗死心包炎和后期心肌梗死心包炎

早期心肌梗死心包炎通常在 STEMI 后不久发病并且是一过性的。后期心肌梗死心包炎（Dressler 综合征）典型发病是在 STEMI 后 1～2 周，目前推测其发病机制为心肌坏死对心包的损伤触发免疫介导的病理反应。PPCI 时代早期和后期心肌梗死心包炎都已少见，多见于再灌注延迟、失败以及大面积心肌梗死。心肌梗死心包炎的诊断标准与其他急性心包炎相同，包括：①胸膜炎性胸痛（占 85%～90%）；②心包摩擦音（发生率≤33%）；③ECG 改变（发生率≤60%），表现为急性期新发广泛导联 ST 段抬高（多为轻度和进行性抬高）或者 PR 压低；④心包积液（发生率≤60%），通常较为轻微。符合其中 2 项可以诊断。

STEMI 后心包炎的治疗同心脏损伤后综合征，建议进行抗感染治疗以缓解症状、减少复发。STEMI 后心包炎建议遵照 ESC2015 年版《心包疾病诊断与治疗指南》，首选阿司匹林抗感染治疗。建议剂量为 500～1000mg，每 6～8 小时 1 次，持续 1～2 周，每隔 1～2 周减少日剂量 250～500mg。作为阿司匹林（非甾体类抗炎药物）的辅助，秋水仙碱也是一线药物，建议服用 3 个月。复发性心包炎时建议服用 6 个月。糖皮质激素有使瘢痕组织变薄导致室壁瘤或心脏破裂的风险，因而不建议使用。除非发生血流动力学损害伴有心脏压塞表现，心肌梗死心包炎很少需要心包穿刺。

2. 心包积液

STEMI 后发生心包积液符合心包炎诊断标准时需按照心包炎进行治疗。没有炎症体征而出现全心包积液＞10mm 或者出现怀疑心脏压塞症状时，应当进行超声心动图检查评价是否存在亚急性心脏破裂。超声心动图结论不明确时，应进行心脏磁共振检查。超声心动图可以对积液量进行定量。心包积液如果为血性积液并且再次迅速增多，建议进行探查手术。

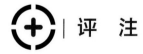 评 注

本章讨论的 STEMI 的并发症包括心肌功能紊乱、心力衰竭、心脏传导异常、心脏机械性并发症和心包炎。在第五章评注中，已经对有些问题进行了评注（请参阅）。

新近发表美国和欧洲心力衰竭指南详述了心力衰竭的处理。对于心源性休克的处理，国内的手段有限。要认识到应用 IABP 主要是增加 STEMI 患者冠状动脉灌注压，改善冠状动脉血流，但是前提是要及早开通梗死相关动脉。IABP 对于改善 STEMI 患者心功能的价值有限。总之，处理 STEMI 的并发症往往需要多学科合作，需要临床医师具备比较全面的知识。

第九章 ⊕
无冠状动脉阻塞的心肌梗死

相当大比例的心肌梗死发生于非阻塞性（狭窄程度＞50%）冠状动脉疾病，发生率1%～14%。临床表现提示心肌缺血和ST段抬高或等同于ST段抬高的患者，即使证明为非阻塞性冠状动脉疾病，也并不能除外病因是冠状动脉粥样硬化血栓形成。因为血栓形成是一个非常动态的过程，其基础的动脉粥样硬化斑块可以是非阻塞性的。

非阻塞性冠状动脉心肌梗死（MINOCA）的诊断标准如表9-1所示。MINOCA是一个诊断过程，经治医师应当寻找潜在的病因。如不能明确病因，会导致患者不能得到充分和恰当的治疗。

表 9-1　非阻塞性冠状动脉心肌梗死的诊断标准（据 Agewalll 等改编）

MINOCA 的诊断依据有 AMI 特征表现患者的冠状动脉造影即刻结果。具体诊断标准如下：
（1）符合全球 AMI 诊断标准
（2）冠状动脉造影未见阻塞病变，即任何可能的梗死相关动脉均无≥50% 的狭窄
（3）没有其他明确临床病因可以解释患者急性期表现

注：MINOCA：非阻塞性冠状动脉心肌梗死；AMI：急性心肌梗死。

ESC有关规范性文件和相关综述已对MINOCA的病因和病理生理学有深入叙述，本指南中不再赘述。根据全球心肌梗死统一定义，MINOCA患者中1型和2型心肌梗死都有可能发生。许多病因都可导致MINOCA，可分类为：①继发于心外膜冠状动脉疾病（如动脉粥样硬化斑块破裂、溃疡、撕裂、侵蚀及非阻塞性冠主动脉病变或正常冠状动脉的夹层）（1型心肌梗死）；②氧的供需失衡（如冠状动脉痉挛或冠状动脉栓塞）（2型心肌梗死）；③冠状动脉内皮功能障碍（如微血管的痉挛）（2型心肌梗死）；④继发于不累及冠状动脉的心肌疾病（如心肌炎或Takotsubo综合征）。最后2种情况类似心肌梗死表现，但归类为心肌损伤更为适合。应对MINOCA进行病因诊断并予以针对性治疗策略。MINOCA的病因与预后强烈相关，其总体预后严重，1年死亡率大约为3.5%。

为了明确MINOCA的病因，建议在冠状动脉造影检查基础上进行其他诊断性检查（图9-1）。通常STEMI患者在排除阻塞性的冠状动脉疾病病因之后，急性期应

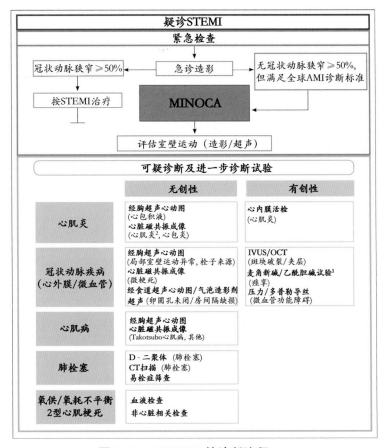

图 9-1　MINOCA 的诊断流程

注：Takotsubo综合征在急性期不能确定诊断，因为根据定义需要影像学随访证实左心室功能恢复。IVUS和OCT较冠状动脉造影往往能够发现更多的动脉粥样硬化斑块。它们也提高了夹层诊断的敏感性。

如果计划进行冠状动脉内影像检查，在急诊心导管检查诊断性冠状动脉造影后实施是适宜的。患者应了解冠状动脉内影像检查可以额外提供更多的信息，但同时也略微增加相关操作风险。

[1] 近期 AMI 可疑有血管痉挛性心绞痛时，可以考虑冠状动脉痉挛激发试验。激发试验必须由有经验的术者进行，而且不一定要在急性期进行。

[2] 临床可疑心肌炎的 ESC 指南编写委员会标准：冠状动脉成像没有 ≥ 50% 狭窄并且 CMR 无心肌缺血表现。确诊心肌炎的 ESC 指南编写委员会标准：冠状动脉成像没有 ≥ 50% 狭窄并且心内膜活检证实 [组织学、免疫组织学、聚合酶链反应技术查找感染病原体（病毒最常见）基因组]。

考虑左心室造影或超声心动图以评估室壁运动和心包积液。此外，如果怀疑上述任一种可能的病因，应当考虑进行其他诊断性检查。

心脏磁共振是一种非常有效的影像技术。因其具有独特的无创评估组织学特征，用来评价室壁运动异常及水肿、心肌瘢痕或纤维化的存在与分布。应当考虑发病 2 周内行磁共振检查，以提高识别 MINOCA 病因的诊断准确性。

⊕ | 评 注

相当比例的 STEMI 患者急诊血管造影并没有严重冠状动脉狭窄，需要进行鉴别诊断和相应的治疗。大约有 14% 的 STEMI 患者"冠状动脉造影正常"，临床多会认为是由于冠状动脉痉挛所致。实际上，冠状动脉走形变异和主动脉疾病累及冠状动脉等，均可以导致"冠状动脉造影正常"，因此应当注意鉴别。

⊕ 第十章
医疗质量评估

全球范围内，STEMI 患者住院期间实际医疗情况和最优化医疗要求之间存在着不小的差距。为了缩小这种差距并且提高医疗质量，建议 STEMI 救治网络和各组成部分建立可评估的质量指标和体系，并对这些指标进行评价与比较、定期审查，保证每个 STEMI 患者都能最大限度获得可行标准所要求的医疗和效果。质量指标的目的是评价和比较卫生服务部门的医疗行为，并为质量改进提供参考。建议用于评估医疗服务质量的指标列于表 10-1。

表 10-1 质量指标

指标或过程类型	质量指标
结构评定（组织）	治疗中心应属于旨在快速有效地提供再灌注治疗的区域网络的一部分，并有书面协议以下涵盖要点：
	·唯一的急救电话号码以便患者呼救联络
	·院前能判读 ECG 结果并做出诊断和将患者运送至 PCI 中心的决定
	·院前启动导管室
	·运送设施（如急救直升机）应配备心电图机、除颤仪
	医疗中心及网络系统人员应详细记录再灌注治疗过程中的关键时间点，并定期进行质量评估审查

续表

指标或过程类型	质量指标
再灌注治疗的质量评估	在发病 12 小时内接受再灌注治疗的 STEMI 患者比例； 及时接受再灌注治疗患者的比例，定义为： · 入院前 · 从诊断到 PCI 再灌注术中导丝通过 IRA 的时间＜ 90min · 从诊断到溶栓再灌注时给予溶栓药物负荷量的时间＜ 10min · 就诊于 PCI 中心的患者 · 从诊断到 PCI 再灌注术中导丝通过 IRA 的时间＜ 60min · 转运患者 · 从诊断到 PCI 再灌注术中导丝通过 IRA 的时间＜ 120min · 就诊于非 PCI 中心的患者门进门出时间＜ 30min（向 PCI 中心运送途中）
住院期间对患者进行风险评价的质量评估	出院前接受 LVEF 评估的患者比例
住院期间患者抗栓治疗的质量评估	无明确阿司匹林和（或）P_2Y_{12} 抑制剂禁忌证，出院时服用 DAPT 患者的比例
出院后患者药物治疗及随诊的质量评估	无他汀禁忌证患者继续按照出院时处方使用他汀类药物（高强度）的比例 无 β - 受体阻滞剂禁忌证且 LVEF ≤ 40% 或心力衰竭患者继续按照出院时处方使用 β - 受体阻滞剂的比例 无 ACEI/ARB 禁忌证且 LVEF ≤ 40% 或心力衰竭患者继续按照出院时处方使用 ACEI（若不能耐受则使用 ARB）的比例 出院时接受戒烟建议和指导的患者比例 无禁忌证患者出院后进行二级预防和心脏康复治疗的比例
患者报告的结果	是否建立一个获取关于患者体验及其所接受信息的质量信息反馈机制，包括以下几点： · 心绞痛的控制 · 医师或护士关于疾病、出院治疗的获益与风险比和医疗随访的解释 · 出院时有关如何应对症状复发和参加心脏康复项目的建议（包括戒烟、饮食咨询）
结果评价	1）校正的 30 天死亡率（如 GRACE 危险评分校正） 2）校正的 30 天再入院率

续表

指标或过程类型	质量指标
机会型复合质量指标	·LVEF > 40% 且无心力衰竭的患者出院后使用低剂量阿司匹林、P_2Y_{12} 抑制剂及高强度他汀类药物的比例 ·LVEF ≤ 40% 和（或）心力衰竭的患者出院后使用低剂量阿司匹林、P_2Y_{12} 抑制剂及高强度他汀类药物、ACEI（或 ARB）及 β - 受体阻滞剂的比例

通常是根据指南的治疗建议进行绩效评估。指南确定了针对所有符合条件并没有禁忌证的患者所应享受的最低限度的医疗标准。建议进行多途径质量评价，包括对机构进行评价（结构评估）、关键临床结果的评估（医疗结果）和患者的经验反馈（患者报告的结果）。ESC 的 ACCA 制定并详细论述了针对急性心肌梗死患者医疗质量、标准化处理及质量计划实施情况的核心指标。已有报道显示，医院对这些质量指标的遵从程度和 30 天死亡率呈负相关。为了使这些指标对医疗机构发挥最大限度影响，临床医师、医院和医疗网络需要投入足够的时间和资源来评价其行为对质量指标的影响，并努力改进方案以达到最佳绩效。

地方 STEMI 诊疗机构应当在系统层面上评估本机构的医疗质量，应参与到为迅速有效救治 STEMI 患者而成立的正式的 STEMI 区域救治网络。制定书面的操作手册，内容应包含：①方便患者联络；②有能力根据院前心电图做出快速诊断并立即转运至 PCI 中心；③院前通过一个急诊电话号码启动导管室；④配置适应当地环境和距离的转运设备 [如急救车、直升机和（或）固定翼飞机]，并装备除颤仪。系统参与人员应详细记录关键再灌注时间信息，并接受协调中心的定期质量评估审查。

及时再灌注治疗是 STEMI 治疗的基石。因此，绩效评估应包括发病 12 小时内患者接受再灌注治疗的比例、患者由于进入救治系统（如 EMS、PCI 中心或者非 PCI 中心）的方式不同所获得指南建议的再灌注治疗的速度。应当详细记录时间延迟信息，定期接受审查评价指南建议时间范围内接受 PPCI 患者的比例（STEMI 确诊后 90min 内患者直接到达 PCI 中心时 60min 内导丝通过梗死相关动脉）。需要指出，这些 PPCI 的时间延迟数据是质量控制指标，与 PPCI 最大时间延迟指标不超过 120min 不同。后者用来决定是否优先选择 PPCI 进行再灌注而不是选择溶栓治疗。理想情况下，这些指标应当接受国家水平的审查，然而实际上大多数欧洲国家没有做到。

其他绩效评估包括患者接受以下措施的比例：在住院期间接受适当种类 P_2Y_{12} 受体拮抗剂、强化他汀治疗、β - 受体阻滞剂、LVEF ≤ 40% 或临床有心力衰竭证据的患者出院前服用 ACEI、出院前戒烟咨询和建议加入二级预防和（或）心脏康复计划。把患者临床结果作为一项质量指标是有争议的。因为许多因素可以影响预后，如死亡率，但是它与质量没有关系（如年龄和最初临床状况）。但是，对主要临床结果进行分析，如 30 天风险校正的死亡率和再住院率，有助于从全球高度观察系统的质量情况，指出需要改进医疗质量的方面，尤其当发现不同中心之间存在明显治疗差异时。最后，需要考虑患者方面因素。应纳入以下指标：针对患者疼痛的处理，因病住院期间医护对病情和治疗措施获益与风险的解释，出院前提供关于自理及生活方式的建议（包括戒烟和饮食咨询）、康复计划、二级预防药物及医学随访等信息的质量和准确性。这些都可能有利于提高全球医疗服务的质量。

机会型复合质量指标分析不同质量指标体系呈"全或无"反应。对于 STEMI 患者，复合质量指标即适合于 LVEF > 40% 并且没有心力衰竭表现的患者（接受低剂量的阿司匹林、P_2Y_{12} 受体拮抗剂和高强度他汀治疗），也适合于 LVEF ≤ 40% 和（或）有心力衰竭临床证据的患者（前者基础上加用 ACEI 或 ARB 和 β - 受体阻滞剂）。已有研究在不同人群中分析了这些复合质量指标与急性心肌梗死后死亡率的关系。

⊕ | 评　注

某些情况下，以指南为基础的优化治疗与 STEMI 患者实际治疗之间存在差距。为了缩小差距，要建立良好的质控体系来改善临床实践结果。没有质控的体系不是好的体系。建立良好的质控标准，定期评估 STEMI 救治体系，是提高救治体系质量的关键。中国在这方面还有很长的路要走。

第十一章
缺乏证据和将来研究的领域

尽管最近几十年 STEMI 的诊治取得了巨大进步，但仍存在着很多重要的不明确的领域，需要在未来进一步探索。在此，我们讨论其中一些未来几年亟待回答的问题。

1. 公共意识和急诊医疗

STEMI 的极早期最容易发生心源性猝死，因而是最有危险的时期。因此，在公众教育健康宣教时应当明确指出，发生心肌缺血症状时最安全的呼救方式就是呼叫 EMS。一些中心和地区已在构建介入团队的日常预警机制和高质量快速救治 STEMI 体制方面取得了巨大的进步。然而，在全球范围内，包括农村地区，院前和院内的处理还有很大差异，有必要进行统一。教育计划和跨国交换专家对此会有帮助。

目前将诊断 STEMI 到预计 PCI 介导的再灌注治疗的时间延迟 120min 作为选择 PCI 术或者溶栓治疗的界值，是基于相对较为陈旧的注册研究和临床试验结果得出的。这些研究往往采用了不同的治疗策略。因此，确定时间延迟最佳界值以指导再灌注策略选择至关重要。

2. 减轻缺血 / 再灌注损伤

心肌梗死面积是 STEMI 幸存者远期不良事件发生的最强预测因素之一。因此，在临床中确立一项减少心肌梗死面积的治疗方法会产生巨大的临床和社会经济学影响。一些实验研究和小规模临床试验显示，某些药物和器械治疗措施可以通过减轻缺血 /

再灌注损伤（包括微血管阻塞）而限制心肌梗死面积。然而，目前还没有大型临床试验证实其临床获益。其中一个原因可能是难以筹措到足够的科研经费来进行大型临床试验以验证其效果。

3. 急性期和长期抗栓药物治疗方案的优化

抗栓治疗是 STEMI 药物治疗的基石。尽管当前已取得了巨大进步，还有一些重要的问题没有解决。对于有口服抗凝指征的患者，最佳的急性期及维持期抗栓治疗策略是什么？口服负荷剂量 P_2Y_{12} 抑制剂的最佳时机和最佳静脉抗栓药物策略是什么？溶栓治疗的患者使用强效 P_2Y_{12} 抑制剂的效果如何？阿司匹林在使用强效抗血小板药物和低剂量抗凝药物的新时期的真实地位如何？ P_2Y_{12} 抑制剂作为单药或联合用药维持抗栓时的最佳服用期限有多长？

4. β - 受体阻滞剂和 ACEI

尽管几十年来关于此类药物的研究已非常深入，但直到最近依然缺乏足够有说服力的临床试验。β - 受体阻滞剂的最佳启动时间（和服药途径）还不清楚。长期维持服用 β - 受体阻滞剂对于心力衰竭和（或）低 LVEF 患者的作用是明确的，但是对于接受再灌注治疗的 STEMI 患者的临床价值还没有前瞻性临床试验证实。长期维持服用 ACEI 类药物也面临同样的问题。

5. STEMI 后风险分层

STEMI 急性期和早期发生过室速或室颤的患者，降低其猝死风险的最佳治疗策略仍不是十分清楚。STEMI 后数周低 LVEF 和低心功能分级的患者置入埋藏式心律转复除颤器有明确的临床获益，但是还需要建立更好的猝死风险分层方法。

非梗死相关动脉病变的最佳处理方案需要确立。有待回答问题包括：指导 PCI 的最佳标准（造影、FFR 或斑块易损性评估）；完全血运重建的最佳时机，一次完成还是分次完成 PCI（包括住院期间和出院后的比较）。

6. 休克和左心室辅助装置

严重心力衰竭和休克是 STEMI 患者最重要的不良预后预测因素。除了紧急梗死相关动脉血运重建以及降低前后负荷的标准药物治疗外，并没有充分的证据证明外周使用正性肌力和血管收缩药以及机械辅助装置的有效性。同样，常规于 PPCI 术中进行完全血运重建的获益也未得到正式证明。IABP 的使用也并未带来预期的临床获益。左心辅助装置和 ECMO 使用越来越广泛，但尚未得到临床试验的充分评估。迫切需要对休克患者使用药物、介入治疗和左室辅助装置效果进行系统性评估研究。

7. 心肌修复 / 补救

新型治疗措施（例如细胞治疗或基因治疗）替代死亡的心肌或者预防不良心室重构的有效性还没有确立。应大力支持基础研究进一步了解心肌发生和修复的生物学过程，为实现基础研究成果向临床相关动物模型的转化乃至最终临床应用提供充分的理论支持。

8. 观察性数据和真实世界证据的需求

为了更好地理解临床实践中存在的缺陷和挑战，需要建立未经筛选但获得认证的注册研究和临床数据库以进行质量评估和标准化处理。在这份文件中，我们指定了质量指标用来评价和比较部门之间卫生服务的质量，并作为质量改进措施的依据。这些质量指标对手术操作和临床结果的影响还有待评估。

9. 实用性临床试验的需求

高度选择性的临床对照试验的一个主要局限就是其在真实世界的适用性。入选标准严格、定制化处理并且随访时间短暂均可导致偏倚，因而妨碍其广泛应用。可以推行实用性临床试验包括基于注册的随机临床试验。这些临床试验入选的选择性低，也没有传统临床试验昂贵，尤其适用于验证治疗措施在临床实践中的效果。

第十二章
本指南要点

1. STEMI 的流行病学

虽然过去几十年欧洲缺血性心脏病死亡率已有下降，缺血性心脏病在世界范围内仍然是最常见的死因。STEMI 和 NSTEMI 的相对发病率分别呈下降和增加趋势。随着再灌注治疗的推广，STEMI 的急性期和远期死亡率下降。然而，STEMI 的死亡率问题依然严峻。ESC 国家注册数据显示真实世界 STEMI 患者的住院死亡率为 4% ~ 12%。

2. 性别问题

与男性相比，女性有更少和（或）更迟的接受再灌注治疗和循证治疗的倾向。需要强调，女性和男性从再灌注和其他 STEMI 相关的治疗中的获益是相同的，因此，针对男性和女性患者应当给予同等的处理。

3. 心电图和 STEMI 诊断

在某些情况下，冠状动脉闭塞和（或）全心缺血可能不伴有特征性 ST 段抬高 [如束支传导阻滞，心室起搏，超急性期 T 波，前壁导联孤立性 ST 段压低和（或）广泛导联 ST 段下压同时伴有 aVR 导联 ST 段抬高]。除非估计从 STEMI 诊断时间开始到 PCI 再灌注的绝对时间长度＞ 120min，当患者出现上述心电图改变伴有符合进行性心肌缺血的临床表现时，应启动 PPCI 策略 （即紧急冠状动脉造影并在有指征时 PCI）。

4. 再灌注策略的选择

STEMI 诊断（指有缺血症状患者的心电图判读发现有 ST 段抬高或等同改变）的时间点就是再灌注策略计时的开始。除非从 STEMI 诊断到 PCI 介导的再灌注耗时间预计＞120min，对 STEMI 患者应当采取 PPCI 策略。否则应立即开始溶栓治疗（STEMI 诊断后的 10min 以内）。

5. STEMI 救治网络

医院和 EMS 之间签署书面协议开展协作在 STEMI 的处理中处于核心地位。不论是 PPCI 策略还是院前溶栓策略，EMS 应当运送患者到 24 小时 7 天不间断开放的高容量的 PCI 中心。在选择再灌注策略后，EMS 应当总是立即通知 PCI 中心。运送患者到 PCI 中心时应绕过急诊室。

6. 心脏骤停和再灌注策略

复苏后的患者心电图有 ST 段抬高时，应采取 PPCI 策略。复苏后心电图没有 ST 段抬高，但高度怀疑有进行性心肌缺血时，在快速评估排除非冠状动脉的原因后，应在 2 小时内进行紧急的冠状动脉造影。做紧急冠状动脉造影决策时应当顾及与神经系统不良后果相关的因素。

7. PPCI 的技术问题

经桡动脉途径和常规置入药物洗脱支架是 PPCI 的标准治疗。禁忌常规血栓抽吸或延迟置入支架策略。

8. 非梗死相关动脉的处理

非梗死相关动脉的严重狭窄（血管造影或 FFR 评估）应当在出院前予以处理（可以在 PPCI 时同期或 PPCI 后分次处理）。心源性休克时应当考虑在 PPCI 时同期进行非梗死相关动脉的 PCI。

9. 抗栓治疗

抗凝和 DAPT 是 STEMI 急性期药物治疗的基石。PPCI：普通肝素（也可以使用依诺肝素或比伐卢定）、负荷剂量阿司匹林和普拉格雷（或替格瑞洛）。溶栓治疗：依诺肝素（也可以使用普通肝素）、负荷剂量阿司匹林和氯吡格雷。大多数患者的维持治疗是 DAPT，即阿司匹林联合普拉格雷（或替格瑞洛）1 年。

10. 早期治疗

再灌注治疗后应对患者进行监测至少 24 小时。没有并发症的患者最好早期下床活动和早期出院。不过，这会导致实施二级预防的时间有限。因此，强调所有相关人员之间进行密切合作十分重要。

11. 特殊患者

强化抗栓治疗在口服抗凝药的肾功能不全和（或）老年患者面临挑战。对这些患者要特别注意某些药物在使用时应进行剂量调整。糖尿病和没有接受再灌注治疗的患者也有特殊性，应予以关注。

12. STEMI 影像评估

无创影像技术在 STEMI 患者的急性期和远期处理中具有重要价值。

13. MINOCA

有相当一部分 STEMI 患者紧急冠状动脉造影时发现没有明显的冠状动脉狭窄。对这些患者应进行其他诊断性检查，查找病因并有针对性地调整治疗方案。

14. 质量指标

有时，某些 STEMI 患者的实际治疗方案同指南建议的最佳治疗方案之间存在差距。为了缩小差距，重要的是在真实世界临床实践中对已确立的质量指标进行评价，以便指导并改进临床实践。建议采用明确定义和经过验证的质量指标来评价和提高 STEMI 治疗水平。

第十三章 ⊕
重要建议小结

重要建议小结见表 13-1。

表 13-1　重要建议小结

建议	建议分类	证据水平
初步诊断		
FMC 后尽快行 12 导联心电图检查和判读，最迟不超过 10min	I	B
所有可疑 STEMI 的患者均尽快使用心电除颤监护仪进行监测	I	B
改善低氧血症和症状		
不建议 SaO$_2$ ≥ 90% 的患者常规吸氧	III	B
心脏骤停的建议		
心脏骤停复苏后心电图提示 STEMI 的患者建议实施 PPCI	I	B
心脏骤停心肺复苏后仍无反应的患者早期进行目标化体温处理	I	B
不建议在院前对自主循环恢复后的患者立即快速输注大量低温液体降低体温	III	B
院前急救调度		
应依靠旨在快速有效地提供再灌注治疗的区域网络对 STEMI 患者进行院前救治，为尽可能多的患者实施 PPCI	I	B
有 PPCI 能力的医疗中心应提供 24 小时 7 天不间断服务，并且能够毫不延迟地实施 PPCI	I	B
患者转运到具有 PCI 能力的中心时应当绕过急诊室和冠心病监护病房（或心脏重症监护病房），直接送达导管室	I	B

建议	建议分类	证据水平
再灌注治疗		
所有缺血症状持续时间 ≤ 12 小时并且 ST 段持续抬高的患者都应实施再灌注治疗	I	A
如果在 STEMI 诊断后不能及时实施 PPCI，建议对症状发作在 12 小时以内并且没有禁忌证的患者进行溶栓治疗	I	A
STEMI 发病超过 48 小时且没有症状患者，不建议对其闭塞梗死相关动脉常规实施 PCI	III	A
PPCI 技术操作问题		
建议对梗死相关动脉实施 PPCI	I	A
PPCI 时应置入支架，优于球囊扩张血管成形术	I	A
建议 PPCI 术应使用新一代药物洗脱支架，优于使用金属裸支架	I	A
建议桡动脉途径操作熟练的术者实施 PPCI 术时采用桡动脉途径，优于股动脉途径	I	A
不建议常规进行血栓抽吸	III	A
不建议常规延迟支架置入	III	B
PPCI 患者的围术期和术后抗栓治疗		
除非有禁忌证（如高危出血风险），建议在 PCI 术前或者至少在 PCI 时服用强效 P_2Y_{12} 抑制剂（普拉格雷或替格瑞洛）或者氯吡格雷（普拉格雷或替格瑞洛没药或对其有禁忌证时），并且维持服用超过 12 个月	I	A
建议所有患者在无禁忌证时尽快口服或静脉推注（不能吞咽时）阿司匹林	I	B
不建议磺达肝癸钠用于 PPCI 术中抗凝	III	B
溶栓治疗		
当溶栓作为再灌注治疗措施时，建议在 STEMI 诊断后尽快实施，最好在院前进行	I	A
建议使用纤维蛋白特异性药物（替奈普酶、阿替普酶和瑞替普酶）	I	B
建议口服或静脉使用阿司匹林	I	B
建议氯吡格雷联合阿司匹林	I	A
接受溶栓的患者建议使用抗凝治疗，直到血运重建（如果实施）或者到住院第 8 天。抗凝药可以是：	I	A
依诺肝素：静脉推注继之以皮下注射（优于普通肝素）	I	A
普通肝素：根据体重调整剂量，静脉推注负荷量继之以静脉输注	I	B

续表

建议	建议分类	证据水平
建议溶栓后立即将患者转运至有 PCI 能力的中心	I	A
对于心力衰竭或休克患者建议行急诊冠状动脉造影，有指征时行 PCI	I	A
当溶栓失败（60 ～ 90min 时 ST 段回落＜ 50%）、出现血流动力学或者心电活动不稳定，或心肌缺血加重时均建议行补救性 PCI	I	A
建议在溶栓成功后 2 ～ 24 小时进行冠状动脉造影，如有指征对梗死相关动脉实施 PCI	I	A
溶栓成功后再发心肌缺血或有证据提示血管再闭塞时，建议行急诊冠状动脉造影，必要时行 PCI	I	B

STEMI 患者的影像学检查和负荷试验

建议住院期间所有 STEMI 患者常规进行超声心动图检查，以评估静息状态下左心室和右心室功能，检查心肌梗死早期机械并发症并排除左心室血栓形成	I	B

STEMI 后的生活方式

建议确定患者是否吸烟。反复建议吸烟患者戒烟，通过随访支持、尼古丁替代治疗、伐尼克兰和安非他酮等方法单用或联用帮助其戒烟	I	A
建议患者参与心脏康复治疗	I	A

STEMI 后的维持抗栓策略

建议低剂量阿司匹林（75 ～ 100mg）抗血小板治疗	I	A
除非有禁忌证（如高危出血风险），建议 PCI 术后 DAPT 方案 12 个月，采用阿司匹林联合替格瑞洛或普拉格雷（普拉格雷或替格瑞洛没药或对其有禁忌证时使用氯吡格雷）	I	A
有高危胃肠道出血风险患者建议质子泵抑制剂（PPI）联合 DAPT 治疗	I	B

急性期、亚急性期和长期常规治疗

除非有禁忌证，心力衰竭和（或）LVEF ≤ 40% 的患者应口服 β - 受体阻滞剂	I	A
低血压、急性心力衰竭、房室传导阻滞和严重心动过缓患者应避免静脉使用 β - 受体阻滞剂	III	B
除非有禁忌证，建议尽早启动强化他汀治疗并长期维持	I	A
目标 LDL-C 水平＜ 1.8mmol/L（70mg/dl），或者 LDL-C 基线水平在 1.8 ～ 3.5mmol/L（70 ～ 135mg/dl）的患者至少降低 50%	I	B
建议 STEMI 合并心力衰竭、左室收缩功能不全、糖尿病或前壁心肌梗死患者在 24 小时内启动 ACEI 治疗	I	A

建议	建议分类	证据水平
合并心力衰竭和（或）左心室收缩功能不全患者可以使用 ARB（优选缬沙坦）替代 ACEI，尤其是患者不能耐受 ACEI 时	I	B
若无肾衰竭或高钾血症，建议 LVEF ≤ 40% 同时有心力衰竭或糖尿病的患者在已经使用 ACEI 和 β-受体阻滞剂基础上服用盐皮质激素受体拮抗剂	I	B

STEMI 后左室功能不全和急性心力衰竭的处理

建议 LVEF ≤ 40% 和（或）心力衰竭患者在血流动力学稳定后尽早使用 ACEI（若不能耐受则使用 ARB），以减少住院和死亡风险	I	A
建议 LVEF ≤ 40% 和（或）心力衰竭患者稳定后使用 β-受体阻滞剂，以减少死亡、再发心肌梗死及因心力衰竭再住院风险	I	A
若无严重肾功能不全和高钾血症，建议心力衰竭并且 LVEF ≤ 40% 的患者使用盐皮质激素受体拮抗剂，以减少心血管再住院和死亡风险	I	B

STEMI 心源性休克的处理

心源性休克患者若冠状动脉解剖适宜，建议即刻实施 PCI。如果冠状动脉解剖不适宜 PCI 术或 PCI 术失败，建议行急诊 CABG	I	B
不建议常规使用 IABP	Ⅲ	B

房颤的处理

地高辛对转复新发房颤无效，也不建议其用于节律控制	Ⅲ	A
钙拮抗药和 β-受体阻滞剂包括索他洛尔对转复新发房颤无效	Ⅲ	B
不建议预防性使用抗心律失常药物预防房颤	Ⅲ	B

心肌梗死急性期室性心律失常和传导系统异常的处理

除非有禁忌证，对于多形性室速和（或）室颤患者建议静脉使用 β-受体阻滞剂	I	B
不建议预防性使用抗心律失常药物，可能有害	Ⅲ	B

室性心律失常的长期处理及猝死风险评估

经过 > 3 个月强化药物治疗并且心肌梗死至少 6 周以后的患者，有症状性心力衰竭（NYHA Ⅱ～Ⅲ级）同时 LVEF ≤ 35%，并且预期寿命 ≥ 1 年时，建议置入埋藏式心律转复除颤器以减少心源性猝死风险	I	A

⊕ 参考文献

[1] Windecker S, Kolh P, Alfonso F, et al.2014 ESC/EACTS Guidelines on myocardial revascularization: the Task Force on Myocardial Revascularization of the European Society of Cardiology (ESC) and the European Association for Cardio-Thoracic Surgery (EACTS). Developed with the special contribution of the European Association of Percutaneous Cardiovascular Interventions (EAPCI). Eur Heart J, 2014, 35 (37): 2541-2619.

[2] Roffi M, Patrono C, Collet JP, et al. 2015 ESC Guidelines for the management of acute coronary syndromesin patients presenting without persistent ST-segment elevation: task Force for the Management of Acute Coronary Syndromes in Patients Presenting without Persistent ST-Segment Elevation of the European Society of Cardiology (ESC). Eur Heart J, 2016, 37 (3): 267-315.

[3] Priori SG, Blomström-Lundqvist C, Mazzanti A, et al. 2015 ESC Guidelines for the management of patients with ventricular arrhythmias and the prevention of sudden cardiac death: the Task Force for the Management of Patients with Ventricular Arrhythmias and the Prevention of Sudden Cardiac Death of the European Society of Cardiology (ESC). Endorsed by: Association for European Paediatric and Congenital Cardiology (AEPC). Eur Heart J, 2015, 36 (41): 2793-2867.

[4] Piepoli MF, Hoes AW, Agewall S, et al. 2016 European Guidelines on cardiovascular disease prevention in clinical practice: the Sixth Joint Task Force of the European Society of Cardiology and Other Societies on Cardiovascular Disease Prevention in Clinical Practice (constituted by representatives of 10 societies and by invited experts). Developed with the special contribution of the European Association for Cardiovascular Prevention & Rehabilitation (EACPR). Eur Heart J, 2016, 37 (29): 2315-2381.

[5] Kirchhof P, Benussi S, Kotecha D, et al. 2016 ESC Guidelines for the management of atrial fibrillation developed in collaboration with EACTS. Eur Heart J, 2016, 37 (38): 2893-2962.

[6] Ponikowski P, Voors AA, Anker SD, et al. 2016 ESC Guidelines for the diagnosis and treatment of acute and chronic heart failure: the Task Force for the diagnosis and treatment of acute and chronic heart failure of the European Society of Cardiology (ESC). Developed with the special contribution of the Heart Failure Association (HFA) of the ESC. Eur Heart J, 2016, 37 (27): 2129-2200.

[7] Valgimigli M, Bueno H, Byrne RA, et al. 2017 ESC focused update on dual antiplatelet therapy in coronary artery disease developed in collaboration with EACTS: the Task Force for dual antiplatelet therapy in coronary artery disease of the European Society of Cardiology (ESC) and of the European Association for Cardio-Thoracic Surgery (EACTS). Eur Heart J, 2018, 39 (3): 213-260.

[8] Thygesen K, Alpert JS, Jaffe AS, et al. Third universal definition of myocardial infarction. Eur Heart J, 2012, 33 (20): 2551-2567.

[9] Gehrie ER, Reynolds HR, Chen AY, et al. Characterization and outcomes of women and men with non-ST-segment elevation myocardial infarction and nonobstructive coronary artery disease: results from the Can Rapid Risk Stratification of Unstable Angina Patients Suppress Adverse Outcomes with Early Implementation of the ACC/AHA Guidelines (CRUSADE) quality improvement initiative. Am Heart J, 2009, 158 (4): 688-694.

[10] Pasupathy S, Air T, Dreyer RP, et al. Systematic review of patients presenting with suspected myocardial infarction and nonobstructive coronary arteries. Circulation, 2015, 131 (10): 861-870.

[11] Niccoli G, Scalone G, Crea F. Acute myocardial infarction with no obstructive coronary atherosclerosis: mechanisms and management. Eur Heart J, 2015, 36 (8): 475-481.

[12] Agewall S, Beltrame JF, Reynolds HR, et al. ESC working group position paper on myocardial infarction with non-obstructive coronary arteries. Eur Heart J, 2017, 38 (3): 143-153.

[13] Hartley A, Marshall DC, Salciccioli JD, et al. Trends in mortality from ischemic heart disease and cerebrovascular disease in Europe: 1980 to 2009. Circulation, 2016, 133 (20): 1916-1926.

[14] Townsend N, Wilson L, Bhatnagar P, et al. Cardiovascular disease in Europe: epidemiological update 2016. Eur Heart J, 2016, 37 (42): 3232-3245.

[15] Sugiyama T, Hasegawa K, Kobayashi Y, et al. Differential time trends of outcomes and costs of care for acute myocardial infarction hospitalizations by ST elevation and type of intervention in the United States, 2001-2011. J Am Heart Assoc, 2015, 4 (3): e001445.

[16] McManus DD, Gore J, Yarzebski J, et al. Recent trends in the incidence, treatment, and outcomes of patients with STEMI and NSTEMI. Am J Med, 2011, 124 (1): 40-47.

[17] Jernberg T. Swede heart Annual Report 2015//Karolinska University Hospital, Huddinge, 14186 Stockholm, 2016.

[18] Widimsky P, Wijns W, Fajadet J, et al. Reperfusion therapy for ST elevation acute myocardial infarction in Europe: description of the current situation in 30 countries. Eur Heart J, 2010, 31 (8): 943-957.

[19] Mozaffarian D, Benjamin EJ, Go AS, et al. Heart disease and stroke statistics—2015 update: a report from the American Heart Association. Circulation, 2015, 131 (4): e29-322.

[20] Khera S, Kolte D, Gupta T, et al. Temporal trends and sex differences in revascularization and outcomes of ST-segment elevation myocardial infarction in younger adults in the United States. J Am Coll Cardiol, 2015, 66 (18): 1961-1972.

[21] Puymirat E, Simon T, Steg PG, et al. Association of changes in clinical characteristics and management with improvement in survival among patients with ST-elevation myocardial infarction. JAMA, 2012, 308 (10): 998-1006.

[22] Gale CP, Allan V, Cattle BA, et al. Trends in hospital treatments, including revascularisation, following acute myocardial infarction, 2003-2010: a multilevel and relative survival analysis for the National Institute for Cardiovascular Outcomes Research (NICOR). Heart, 2014, 100 (7): 582-589.

[23] Kristensen SD, Laut KG, Fajadet J, et al. Reperfusion therapy for ST elevation acute myocardial infarction 2010/2011: current status in 37 ESC countries. Eur Heart J, 2014, 35 (29): 1957-1970.

[24] Pedersen F, Butrymovich V, Kelbaek H, et al. Short- and long-term cause of death in patients treated with primary PCI for STEMI. J Am Coll Cardiol, 2014, 64 (20): 2101-2108.

[25] Fokkema ML, James SK, Albertsson P, et al. Population trends in percutaneous coronary intervention: 20-year results from the SCAAR (Swedish Coronary Angiography and Angioplasty Registry). J Am Coll Cardiol, 2013, 61 (12): 1222-1230.

[26] EUGenMed Cardiovascular Clinical Study Group, Regitz-Zagrosek V, Oertelt- Prigione S, et al. Gender in cardiovascular diseases: impact on clinical manifestations, management, and outcomes. Eur Heart J, 2016, 37 (1): 24-34.

[27] Brieger D, Eagle KA, Goodman SG, et al. Acute coronary syndromes without chest pain, an underdiagnosed and undertreated high-risk group: insights from the Global Registry of Acute Coronary Events. Chest, 2004, 126 (2): 461-469.

[28] Kaul P, Armstrong PW, Sookram S, et al. Temporal trends in patient and treatment delay among men and women presenting with ST-elevation myocardial infarction. Am Heart J, 2011, 161 (1): 91-97.

[29] Diercks DB, Owen KP, Kontos MC, et al. Gender differences in time to presentation for myocardial infarction before and after a national women's cardiovascular awareness campaign: a temporal analysis from the Can Rapid Risk Stratification of Unstable Angina Patients Suppress ADverse Outcomes with Early Implementation (CRUSADE) and the National Cardiovascular Data Registry Acute Coronary Treatment and Intervention Outcomes Network-Get with the Guidelines (NCDR ACTION Registry-GWTG). Am Heart J, 2010, 160 (1): 80-87, e3.

[30] Kang SH, Suh JW, Yoon CH, et al. Sex differences in management and mortality of patients with ST-elevation myocardial infarction (from the Korean Acute Myocardial Infarction National Registry). Am J Cardiol, 2012, 109 (6): 787-793.

[31] Kyto V, Sipila J, Rautava P. Gender and in-hospital mortality of ST-segment elevation myocardial infarction (from a multihospital nationwide registry study of 31689 patients). Am J Cardiol, 2015, 115 (3): 303-306.

[32] Hvelplund A, Galatius S, Madsen M, et al. Women with acute coronary syndrome are less invasively examined and subsequently less treated than men. Eur Heart J, 2010, 31 (6): 684-690.

[33] Nguyen JT, Berger AK, Duval S, et al. Gender disparity in cardiac procedures and medication use for acute myocardial infarction. Am Heart J, 2008, 155 (5): 862-868.

[34] De Torbal A, Boersma E, Kors JA, et al. Incidence of recognized and unrecognized myocardial infarction in men and women aged 55 and older: the Rotterdam Study. Eur Heart J, 2006, 27 (6): 729-736.

[35] Henrikson CA, Howell EE, Bush DE, et al. Chest pain relief by nitroglycerin does not predict

active coronary artery disease. Ann Intern Med, 2003, 139 (12): 979-986.

[36] Diercks DB, Peacock WF, Hiestand BC, et al. Frequency and consequences of recording an electrocardiogram >10 minutes after arrival in an emergency room in non-ST-segment elevation acute coronary syndromes (from the CRUSADE Initiative). Am J Cardiol, 2006, 97 (4): 437-442.

[37] Tubaro M, Danchin N, Goldstein P, et al. Pre-hospital treatment of STEMI patients. A scientific statement of the Working Group Acute Cardiac Care of the European Society of Cardiology. Acute Card Care, 2011, 13 (2): 56-67.

[38] Rokos IC, French WJ, Koenig WJ, et al. Integration of pre-hospital electrocardiograms and ST-elevation myocardial infarction receiving center (SRC) networks: impact on door-to-balloon times across 10 independent regions. JACC Cardiovasc Interv, 2009, 2 (4): 339-346.

[39] Quinn T, Johnsen S, Gale CP, et al. Effects of prehospital 12-lead ECG on processes of care and mortality in acute coronary syndrome: a linked cohort study from the Myocardial Ischaemia National Audit Project. Heart, 2014, 100 (12): 944-950.

[40] Sorensen JT, Terkelsen CJ, Norgaard BL, et al. Urban and rural implementation of pre-hospital diagnosis and direct referral for primary percutaneous coronary intervention in patients with acute ST-elevation myocardial infarction. Eur Heart J, 2011, 32 (4): 430-436.

[41] Chan AW, Kornder J, Elliott H, et al. Improved survival associated with pre-hospital triage strategy in a large regional ST-segment elevation myocardial infarction program. JACC Cardiovasc Interv, 2012, 5 (12): 1239-1246.

[42] Dhruva VN, Abdelhadi SI, Anis A, et al. ST-Segment Analysis Using Wireless Technology in Acute Myocardial Infarction (STAT-MI) trial. J Am Coll Cardiol, 2007, 50 (6): 509-513.

[43] Lopez-Sendon J, Coma-Canella I, Alcasena S, et al. Electrocardiographic findings in acute right ventricular infarction: sensitivity and specificity of electrocardiographic alterations in right precordial leads V4R, V3R, V1, V2, and V3. J Am Coll Cardiol, 1985, 6 (6): 1273-1279.

[44] O'Doherty M, Tayler DI, Quinn E, et al. Five hundred patients with myocardial infarction monitored within one hour of symptoms. Br Med J (Clin Res Ed) , 1983, 286 (6375): 1405-1408.

[45] Mehta RH, Starr AZ, Lopes RD, et al. Incidence of and outcomes associated with ventricular tachycardia or fibrillation in patients undergoing primary percutaneous coronary intervention.

JAMA, 2009, 301 (17): 1779-1789.

[46] Rokos IC, Farkouh ME, Reiffel J, et al. Correlation between index electrocardiographic patterns and pre-intervention angiographic findings: insights from the HORIZONS-AMI trial. Catheter Cardiovasc Interv, 2012, 79 (7): 1092-1098.

[47] Stribling WK, Kontos MC, Abbate A, et al. Left circumflex occlusion in acute myocardial infarction (from the National Cardiovascular Data Registry). Am J Cardiol, 2011, 108 (7): 959-963.

[48] Dixon WC 4th, Wang TY, Dai D, et al. Anatomic distribution of the culprit lesion in patients with non-ST-segment elevation myocardial infarction undergoing percutaneous coronary intervention: findings from the National Cardiovascular Data Registry. J Am Coll Cardiol, 2008, 52 (16): 1347-1348.

[49] Wang TY, Zhang M, Fu Y, et al. Incidence, distribution, and prognostic impact of occluded culprit arteries among patients with non-STelevation acute coronary syndromes undergoing diagnostic angiography. Am Heart J, 2009, 157 (4): 716-723.

[50] Sgarbossa EB, Pinski SL, Barbagelata A, et al. Electrocardiographic diagnosis of evolving acute myocardial infarction in the presence of left bundle-branch block. GUSTO-1 (Global Utilization of Streptokinase and Tissue Plasminogen Activator for Occluded Coronary Arteries) Investigators. N Engl J Med, 1996, 334 (8): 481-487.

[51] Wong CK, French JK, Aylward PE, et al. Patients with prolonged ischemic chest pain and presumed-new left bundle branch block have heterogeneous outcomes depending on the presence of ST-segment changes. J Am Coll Cardiol, 2005, 46 (1): 29-38.

[52] Shlipak MG, Lyons WL, Go AS, et al. Should the electrocardiogram be used to guide therapy for patients with left bundlebranch block and suspected myocardial infarction?JAMA, 1999, 281 (8): 714-719.

[53] Lopes RD, Siha H, Fu Y, et al. Diagnosing acute myocardial infarction in patients with left bundle branch block. Am J Cardiol, 2011, 108 (6): 782-788.

[54] Chang AM, Shofer FS, Tabas JA, et al. Lack of association between left bundle-branch block and acute myocardial infarction in symptomatic ED patients. Am J Emerg Med, 2009, 27 (8): 916-921.

[55] Widimsky P, Rohac F, Stasek J, et al. Primary angioplasty in acute myocardial infarction with

right bundle branch block: should new onset right bundle branch block be added to future guidelines as an indication for reperfusion therapy?Eur Heart J, 2012, 33 (1): 86-95.

[56] Madias JE. The nonspecificity of ST-segment elevation>or=5.0 mm in V1-V3 in the diagnosis of acute myocardial infarction in the presence of ventricular paced rhythm. J Electrocardiol, 2004, 37 (2): 135-139.

[57] Sgarbossa EB, Pinski SL, Gates KB, et al. Early electrocardiographic diagnosis of acute myocardial infarction in the presence of ventricular paced rhythm. GUSTO-I Investigators. Am J Cardiol, 1996, 77 (5): 423-424.

[58] Krishnaswamy A, Lincoff AM, Menon V. Magnitude and consequences of missing the acute infarct-related circumflex artery. Am Heart J, 2009, 158 (5): 706-712.

[59] From AM, Best PJ, Lennon RJ, et al. Acute myocardial infarction due to left circumflex artery occlusion and significance of ST-segment elevation. Am J Cardiol, 2010, 106 (8): 1081-1085.

[60] Yan AT, Yan RT, Kennelly BM, et al. Relationship of ST elevation in lead aVR with angiographic findings and outcome in non-ST elevation acute coronary syndromes. Am Heart J, 2007, 154 (1): 71-78.

[61] Hobl EL, Stimpfl T, Ebner J, et al. Morphine decreases clopidogrel concentrations and effects: a randomized, double-blind, placebo-controlled trial. J Am Coll Cardiol, 2014, 63 (7): 630-635.

[62] Parodi G, Bellandi B, Xanthopoulou I, et al. Morphine is associated with a delayed activity of oral antiplatelet agents in patients with ST-elevation acute myocardial infarction undergoing primary percutaneous coronary intervention. Circ Cardiovasc Interv, 2015, 8 (1): e001593.

[63] Kubica J, Adamski P, Ostrowska M, et al. Morphine delays and attenuates ticagrelor exposure and action in patients with myocardial infarction: the randomized, double-blind, placebo-controlled IMPRESSION trial. Eur Heart J, 2016, 37 (3): 245-252.

[64] Stub D, Smith K, Bernard S, et al. Air versus oxygen in ST-segment-elevation myocardial infarction. Circulation, 2015, 131 (24): 2143-2150.

[65] Cabello JB, Burls A, Emparanza JI, et al. Oxygen therapy for acute myocardial infarction. Cochrane Database Syst Rev, 2013, 8: CD007160.

[66] Hofmann R, James SK, Svensson L, et al. Determination of the role of oxygen in suspected acute myocardial infarction trial. Am Heart J, 2014, 167 (3): 322-328.

[67] Rawles JM, Kenmure AC. Controlled trial of oxygen in uncomplicated myocardial infarction.

BMJ, 1976, 1 (6018): 1121-1123.

[68] Larsen JM, Ravkilde J. Acute coronary angiography in patients resuscitated from out-of-hospital cardiac arrest: a systematic review and meta-analysis. Resuscitation, 2012, 83 (12): 1427-1433.

[69] Garot P, Lefevre T, Eltchaninoff H, et al. Six-month outcome of emergency percutaneous coronary intervention in resuscitated patients after cardiac arrest complicating ST-elevation myocardial infarction. Circulation, 2007, 115 (11): 1354-1362.

[70] Kern KB, Rahman O. Emergent percutaneous coronary intervention for resuscitated victims of out-of-hospital cardiac arrest. Catheter Cardiovasc Interv, 2010, 75 (4): 616-624.

[71] Spaulding CM, Joly LM, Rosenberg A, et al. Immediate coronary angiography in survivors of out-of-hospital cardiac arrest. N Engl J Med, 1997, 336 (23): 1629-1633.

[72] Dumas F, Cariou A, Manzo-Silberman S, et al. Immediate percutaneous coronary intervention is associated with better survival after out-of-hospital cardiac arrest: insights from the PROCAT (Parisian Region Out of hospital Cardiac ArresT) registry. Circ Cardiovasc Interv, 2010, 3 (3): 200-207.

[73] Noc M, Fajadet J, Lassen JF, et al. Invasive coronary treatment strategies for out-of-hospital cardiac arrest: a consensus statement from the European Association for Percutaneous Cardiovascular Interventions (EAPCI) /Stent for LIfe (SFL) groups. EuroIntervention, 2014, 10 (1): 31-37.

[74] Monsieurs KG, Nolan JP, Bossaert LL, et al. European Resuscitation Council Guidelines for Resuscitation 2015: Section 1. Executive summary. Resuscitation, 2015, 95: 1-80.

[75] Reynolds JC, Frisch A, Rittenberger JC, et al. Duration of resuscitation efforts and functional outcome after out-of-hospital cardiac arrest: when should we change to novel therapies?Circulation, 2013, 128 (23): 2488-2494.

[76] Moulaert VR, Verbunt JA, van Heugten CM, et al. Cognitive impairments in survivors of out-of-hospital cardiac arrest: a systematic review. Resuscitation, 2009, 80 (3): 297-305.

[77] Hypothermia after Cardiac Arrest Study Group. Mild therapeutic hypothermia to improve the neurologic outcome after cardiac arrest. N Engl J Med, 2002, 346 (8): 549-556.

[78] Bernard SA, Gray TW, Buist MD, et al. Treatment of comatose survivors of out-of-hospital cardiac arrest with induced hypothermia. N Engl J Med, 2002, 346 (8): 557-563.

[79] Nikolaou NI, Welsford M, Beygui F, et al. Part 5: Acute coronary syndromes: 2015 International Consensus on Cardiopulmonary Resuscitation and Emergency Cardiovascular Care Science with Treatment Recommendations. Resuscitation, 2015, 95: e121-e146.

[80] Belliard G, Catez E, Charron C, et al. Efficacy of therapeutic hypothermia after out-of-hospital cardiac arrest due to ventricular fibrillation. Resuscitation, 2007, 75 (2): 252-259.

[81] Nielsen N, Wetterslev J, Cronberg T, et al. Targeted temperature management at 33 degrees C versus 36 degrees C after cardiac arrest. N Engl J Med, 2013, 369 (23): 2197-2206.

[82] Vaahersalo J, Hiltunen P, Tiainen M, et al. Therapeutic hypothermia after outof- hospital cardiac arrest in Finnish intensive care units: the FINNRESUSCI study. Intensive Care Med, 2013, 39 (5): 826-837.

[83] Penela D, Magaldi M, Fontanals J, et al. Hypothermia in acute coronary syndrome: brain salvage versus stent thrombosis?J Am Coll Cardiol, 2013, 61 (6): 686-687.

[84] Shah N, Chaudhary R, Mehta K, et al. Therapeutic hypothermia and stent thrombosis: a nationwide analysis. JACC Cardiovasc Interv, 2016, 9 (17): 1801-1811.

[85] Garcia-Tejada J, Jurado-Roman A, Rodriguez J, et al. Post-resuscitation electrocardiograms, acute coronary findings and in-hospital prognosis of survivors of out-of-hospital cardiac arrest. Resuscitation, 2014, 85 (9): 1245-1250.

[86] Kim F, Nichol G, Maynard C, et al. Effect of prehospital induction of mild hypothermia on survival and neurological status among adults with cardiac arrest: a randomized clinical trial. JAMA, 2014, 311 (1): 45-52.

[87] Terkelsen CJ, Sorensen JT, Maeng M, et al. System delay and mortality among patients with STEMI treated with primary percutaneous coronary intervention. JAMA, 2010, 304 (7): 763-771.

[88] Fordyce CB, Al-Khalidi HR, Jollis JG, et al. Association of rapid care process implementation on reperfusion times across multiple ST-segment-elevation myocardial infarction networks. Circ Cardiovasc Interv, 2017, 10 (1): e004061.

[89] Stowens JC, Sonnad SS, Rosenbaum RA. Using EMS dispatch to trigger STEMI alerts decreases door-to-balloon times. West J Emerg Med, 2015, 16 (3): 472-480.

[90] Squire BT, Tamayo-Sarver JH, Rashi P, et al. Effect of prehospital cardiac catheterization lab activation on door-to-balloon time, mortality, and false-positive activation. Prehosp Emerg

Care, 2014, 18 (1): 1-8.

[91] Nallamothu BK, Normand SL, Wang Y, et al. Relation between door-to-balloon times and mortality after primary percutaneous coronary intervention over time: a retrospective study. Lancet, 2015, 385 (9973): 1114-1122.

[92] Bagai A, Jollis JG, Dauerman HL, et al. Emergency department bypass for ST-segment-elevation myocardial infarction patients identified with a prehospital electrocardiogram: a report from the American Heart Association Mission: Lifeline program. Circulation, 2013, 128 (4): 352-359.

[93] Wang TY, Nallamothu BK, Krumholz HM, et al. Association of door-in to door-out time with reperfusion delays and outcomes among patients transferred for primary percutaneous coronary intervention. JAMA, 2011, 305 (24): 2540-2547.

[94] Huber K, De Caterina R, Kristensen SD, et al. Pre-hospital reperfusion therapy: a strategy to improve therapeutic outcome in patients with ST-elevation myocardial infarction. Eur Heart J, 2005, 26 (19): 2063-2074.

[95] Welsh RC, Chang W, Goldstein P, et al. Time to treatment and the impact of a physician on prehospital management of acute ST elevation myocardial infarction: insights from the ASSENT-3 PLUS trial. Heart, 2005, 91 (11): 1400-1406.

[96] Bjorklund E, Stenestrand U, Lindbäck J, et al. Pre-hospital thrombolysis delivered by paramedics is associated with reduced time delay and mortality in ambulance-transported real-life patients with ST-elevation myocardial infarction. Eur Heart J, 2006, 27 (10): 1146-1152.

[97] Steg PG, Bonnefoy E, Chabaud S, et al. Impact of time to treatment on mortality after prehospital fibrinolysis or primary angioplasty: data from the CAPTIM randomized clinical trial. Circulation, 2003, 108 (23): 2851-2856.

[98] Bonnefoy E, Steg PG, Boutitie F, et al. Comparison of primary angioplasty and pre-hospital fibrinolysis in acute myocardial infarction (CAPTIM) trial: a 5-year follow-up. Eur Heart J, 2009, 30 (13): 1598-1606.

[99] Danchin N, Coste P, Ferrieres J, et al. Comparison of thrombolysis followed by broad use of percutaneous coronary intervention with primary percutaneous coronary intervention for ST-segment-elevation acute myocardial infarction: data from the french registry on acute ST-elevation myocardial infarction (FAST-MI). Circulation, 2008, 118 (3): 268-276.

[100] Kalla K, Christ G, Karnik R, et al. Implementation of guidelines improves the standard of care: the Viennese registry on reperfusion strategies in ST-elevation myocardial infarction (Vienna STEMI registry). Circulation, 2006, 113 (20): 2398-2405.

[101] Henry TD, Sharkey SW, Burke MN, et al. A regional system to provide timely access to percutaneous coronary intervention for ST-elevation myocardial infarction. Circulation, 2007, 116 (7): 721-728.

[102] Le May MR, So DY, Dionne R, et al. A citywide protocol for primary PCI in ST-segment elevation myocardial infarction. N Engl J Med, 2008, 358 (3): 231-240.

[103] Knot J, Widimsky P, Wijns W, et al. How to set up an effective national primary angioplasty network: lessons learned from five European countries. EuroIntervention, 2009, 5 (3): 299, 301-309.

[104] Nallamothu BK, Krumholz HM, Ko DT, et al. Development of systems of care for ST-elevation myocardial infarction patients: gaps, barriers, and implications. Circulation, 2007, 116 (2): e68-e72.

[105] Rathore SS, Curtis JP, Chen J, et al. Association of door-to-balloon time and mortality in patients admitted to hospital with ST elevation myocardial infarction: national cohort study. BMJ, 2009, 338: b1807.

[106] Nielsen PH, Terkelsen CJ, Nielsen TT, et al. System delay and timing of intervention in acute myocardial infarction (from the Danish Acute Myocardial Infarction-2 [DANAMI-2] trial). Am J Cardiol, 2011, 108 (6): 776-781.

[107] Pinto DS, Kirtane AJ, Nallamothu BK, et al. Hospital delays in reperfusion for ST-elevation myocardial infarction: implications when selecting a reperfusion strategy. Circulation, 2006, 114 (19): 2019-2025.

[108] Widimsky P, Fajadet J, Danchin N, et al. "Stent 4 Life"targeting PCI at all who will benefit the most. A joint project between EAPCI, Euro-PCR, EUCOMED and the ESC Working Group on Acute Cardiac Care. EuroIntervention, 2009, 4 (5): 555-557.

[109] Steg PG, Cambou JP, Goldstein P, et al. Bypassing the emergency room reduces delays and mortality in ST elevation myocardial infarction: the USIC 2000 registry. Heart, 2006, 92 (10): 1378-1383.

[110] Baran KW, Kamrowski KA, Westwater JJ, et al. Very rapid treatment of ST-segment-elevation

myocardial infarction: utilizing prehospital electrocardiograms to bypass the emergency department. Circ Cardiovasc Qual Outcomes, 2010, 3 (4): 431-437.

[111] Thiemann DR, Coresh J, Oetgen WJ, et al. The association between hospital volume and survival after acute myocardial infarction in elderly patients. N Engl J Med, 1999, 340 (21): 1640-1648.

[112] West RM, Cattle BA, Bouyssie M, et al. Impact of hospital proportion and volume on primary percutaneous coronary intervention performance in England and Wales. Eur Heart J, 2011, 32 (6): 706-711.

[113] Zijlstra F, Hoorntje JC, de Boer MJ, et al. Long-term benefit of primary angioplasty as compared with thrombolytic therapy for acute myocardial infarction. N Engl J Med, 1999, 341 (19): 1413-1419.

[114] Keeley EC, Boura JA, Grines CL. Primary angioplasty versus intravenous thrombolytic therapy for acute myocardial infarction: a quantitative review of 23 randomised trials. Lancet, 2003, 361 (9351): 13-20.

[115] Widimsky P, Budesinsky T, Vorac D, et al. Long distance transport for primary angioplasty vs immediate thrombolysis in acute myocardial infarction. Final results of the randomized national multicentre trial—PRAGUE-2. Eur Heart J, 2003, 24 (1): 94-104.

[116] Andersen HR, Nielsen TT, Rasmussen K, et al. A comparison of coronary angioplasty with fibrinolytic therapy in acute myocardial infarction. N Engl J Med, 2003, 349 (8): 733-742.

[117] Nallamothu BK, Bates ER. Percutaneous coronary intervention versus fibrinolytic therapy in acute myocardial infarction: is timing (almost) everything?Am J Cardiol, 2003, 92 (7): 824-826.

[118] Betriu A, Masotti M. Comparison of mortality rates in acute myocardial infarction treated by percutaneous coronary intervention versus fibrinolysis. Am J Cardiol, 2005, 95 (1): 100-101.

[119] Boersma E, Primary Coronary Angioplasty vs Thrombolysis Group. Does time matter?A pooled analysis of randomized clinical trials comparing primary percutaneous coronary intervention and in-hospital fibrinolysis in acute myocardial infarction patients. Eur Heart J, 2006, 27 (7): 779-788.

[120] Pinto DS, Frederick PD, Chakrabarti AK, et al. Benefit of transferring ST-segment-elevation myocardial infarction patients for percutaneous coronary intervention compared with

administration of onsite fibrinolytic declines as delays increase. Circulation, 2011, 124 (23): 2512-2521.

[121] Armstrong PW, Gershlick AH, Goldstein P, et al. Fibrinolysis or primary PCI in ST-segment elevation myocardial infarction. N Engl J Med, 2013, 368 (15): 1379-1387.

[122] Task Force on the management of ST-segment elevationsacute myocardial infarction of the European Society of Cardiology (ESC) , Steg PG, James SK, et al. ESC Guidelines for the management of acute myocardial infarction in patients presenting with ST-segment elevation. Eur Heart J, 2012, 33 (20): 2569-2619.

[123] Morrison LJ, Verbeck PR, McDonald AC, et al. Mortality and prehospital thrombolysis for acute myocardial infarction: a meta-analysis. JAMA, 2000, 283 (20): 2686-2692.

[124] Gershlick AH, Stephens-Lloyd A, Hughes S, et al. Rescue angioplasty after failed thrombolytic therapy for acute myocardial infarction. N Engl J Med, 2005, 353 (26): 2758-2768.

[125] Madan M, Halvorsen S, Di Mario C, et al. Relationship between time to invasive assessment and clinical outcomes of patients undergoing an early invasive strategy after fibrinolysis for ST-segment elevation myocardial infarction: a patient-level analysis of the randomized early routine invasive clinical trials. JACC Cardiovasc Interv, 2015, 8 (1 Pt B): 166-174.

[126] Cantor WJ, Fitchett D, Borgundvaag B, et al. Routine early angioplasty after fibrinolysis for acute myocardial infarction. N Engl J Med, 2009, 360 (26): 2705-2718.

[127] Di Mario C, Dudek D, Piscione F, et al. Immediate angioplasty versus standard therapy with rescue 3 angioplasty after thrombolysis in the Combined Abciximab REteplase Stent Study in Acute Myocardial Infarction (CARESS-in- AMI): an open, prospective, randomised, multicentre trial. Lancet, 2008, 371 (9612): 559-568.

[128] Bohmer E, Hoffmann P, Abdelnoor M, et al. Efficacy and safety of immediate angioplasty versus ischemia-guided management after thrombolysis in acute myocardial infarction in areas with very long transfer distances. Results of the NORDISTEMI (NORwegian study on DIstrict treatment of ST-Elevation Myocardial Infarction). J Am Coll Cardiol, 2010, 55 (2): 102-110.

[129] Borgia F, Goodman SG, Halvorsen S, et al. Early routine percutaneous coronary intervention after fibrinolysis vs. standard therapy in ST-segment elevation myocardial infarction: a meta-

analysis. Eur Heart J, 2010, 31 (17): 2156-2169.

[130] D'Souza SP, Mamas MA, Fraser DG, et al. Routine early coronary angioplasty versus ischaemia-guided angioplasty after thrombolysis in acute ST elevation myocardial infarction: a meta-analysis. Eur Heart J, 2011, 32 (8): 972-982.

[131] Neeland IJ, Kontos MC, de Lemos JA. Evolving considerations in the management of patients with left bundle branch block and suspected myocardial infarction. J Am Coll Cardiol, 2012, 60 (2): 96-105.

[132] Liakopoulos V, Kellerth T, Christensen K. Left bundle branch block and suspected myocardial infarction: does chronicity of the branch block matter?Eur Heart J Acute Cardiovasc Care, 2013, 2 (2): 182-189.

[133] Schomig A, Mehilli J, Antoniucci D, et al. Mechanical reperfusion in patients with acute myocardial infarction presenting more than 12 hours from symptom onset: a randomized controlled trial. JAMA, 2005, 293 (23): 2865-2872.

[134] Ndrepepa G, Kastrati A, Mehilli J, et al. Mechanical reperfusion and long-term mortality in patients with acute myocardial infarction presenting 12 to 48 hours from onset of symptoms. JAMA, 2009, 301 (5): 487-488.

[135] Hochman JS, Lamas GA, Buller CE, et al. Coronary intervention for persistent occlusion after myocardial infarction. N Engl J Med, 2006, 355 (23): 2395-2407.

[136] Menon V, Pearte CA, Buller CE, et al. Lack of benefit from percutaneous intervention of persistently occluded infarct arteries after the acute phase of myocardial infarction is time independent: insights from Occluded Artery Trial. Eur Heart J, 2009, 30 (2): 183-191.

[137] Ioannidis JP, Katritsis DG. Percutaneous coronary intervention for late reperfusion after myocardial infarction in stable patients. Am Heart J, 2007, 154 (6): 1065-1071.

[138] Boersma E, Maas ACP, Deckers JW, et al. Early thrombolytic treatment in acute myocardial infarction: reappraisal of the golden hour. Lancet, 1996, 348 (9030): 771-775.

[139] Cucherat M, Bonnefoy E, Tremeau G. Primary angioplasty versus intravenous thrombolysis for acute myocardial infarction. Cochrane Database Syst Rev, 2003, 3: CD001560.

[140] Dalby M, Bouzamondo A, Lechat P, et al. Transfer for primary angioplasty versus immediate thrombolysis in acute myocardial infarction: a Metaanalysis. Circulation, 2003, 108 (15): 1809-1814.

[141] Gierlotka M, Gasior M, Wilczek K, et al. Reperfusion by primary percutaneous coronary intervention in patients with ST-segment elevation myocardial infarction within 12 to 24 hours of the onset of symptoms (from a prospective national observational study [PL-ACS]). Am J Cardiol, 2011, 107 (4): 501-508.

[142] Busk M, Kaltoft A, Nielsen SS, et al. Infarct size and myocardial salvage after primary angioplasty in patients presenting with symptoms for <12 h vs. 12~72h. Eur Heart J, 2009, 30 (11): 1322-1330.

[143] Valgimigli M, Gagnor A, Calabro P, et al. Radial versus femoral access in patients with acute coronary syndromes undergoing invasive management: a randomised multicentre trial. Lancet, 2015, 385 (9986): 2465-2476.

[144] Jolly SS, Yusuf S, Cairns J, et al. Radial versus femoral access for coronary angiography and intervention in patients with acute coronary syndromes (RIVAL): a randomised, parallel group, multicentre trial. Lancet, 2011, 377 (9775): 1409-1420.

[145] Romagnoli E, Biondi-Zoccai G, Sciahbasi A, et al. Radial versus femoral randomized investigation in ST-segment elevation acute coronary syndrome: the RIFLE-STEACS (Radial Versus Femoral Randomized Investigation in ST-Elevation Acute Coronary Syndrome) study. J Am Coll Cardiol, 2012, 60 (24): 2481-2489.

[146] Nordmann AJ, Hengstler P, Harr T, et al. Clinical outcomes of primary stenting versus balloon angioplasty in patients with myocardial infarction: a meta-analysis of randomized controlled trials. Am J Med, 2004, 116 (4): 253-262.

[147] Stone GW, Grines CL, Cox DA, et al. Comparison of angioplasty with stenting, with or without abciximab, in acute myocardial infarction. N Engl J Med, 2002, 346 (13): 957-966.

[148] Kastrati A, Dibra A, Spaulding C, et al. Meta-analysis of randomized trials on drug-eluting stents vs. bare-Metal stents in patients with acute myocardial infarction. Eur Heart J, 2007, 28 (22): 2706-2713.

[149] Raber L, Kelbaek H, Ostojic M, et al. Effect of biolimus-eluting stents with biodegradable polymer vs bare-Metal stents on cardiovascular events among patients with acute myocardial infarction: the COMFORTABLE AMI randomized trial. JAMA, 2012, 308 (8): 777-787.

[150] Sabate M, Cequier A, Iniguez A, et al. Everolimus-eluting stent versus bare-Metal stent in ST-segment elevation myocardial infarction (EXAMINATION): 1 year results of a randomised

controlled trial. Lancet, 2012, 380 (9852): 1482-1490.

[151] Sabate M, Brugaletta S, Cequier A, et al. Clinical outcomes in patients with STsegment elevation myocardial infarction treated with everolimus-eluting stents versus bare-Metal stents (EXAMINATION): 5-year results of a randomised trial. Lancet, 2016, 387 (10016): 357-366.

[152] Bonaa KH, Mannsverk J, Wiseth R, et al. Drug-eluting or bare-Metal stents for coronary artery disease. N Engl J Med, 2016, 375 (13): 1242-1252.

[153] Carrick D, Oldroyd KG, McEntegart M, et al. A randomized trial of deferred stenting versus immediate stenting to prevent no- or slow-reflow in acute ST-segment elevation myocardial infarction (DEFER-STEMI). J Am Coll Cardiol, 2014, 63 (20): 2088-2098.

[154] Belle L, Motreff P, Mangin L, et al. Comparison of immediate with delayed stenting using the minimalist immediate mechanical intervention approach in acute ST-segment-elevation myocardial infarction: the MIMI Study. Circ Cardiovasc Interv, 2016, 9 (3): e003388.

[155] Kelbaek H, Hofsten DE, Kober L, et al. Deferred versus conventional stent implantation in patients with ST-segment elevation myocardial infarction (DANAMI 3-DEFER): an open-label, randomised controlled trial. Lancet, 2016, 387 (10034): 2199-2206.

[156] Burzotta F, De Vita M, Gu YL, et al. Clinical impact of thrombectomy in acute ST-elevation myocardial infarction: an individual patient-data pooled analysis of 11 trials. Eur Heart J, 2009, 30 (18): 2193-2203.

[157] Frobert O, Lagerqvist B, Olivecrona GK, et al. Thrombus aspiration during STsegment elevation myocardial infarction. N Engl J Med, 2013, 369 (17): 1587-1597.

[158] Lagerqvist B, Frobert O, Olivecrona GK, et al. Outcomes 1 year after thrombus aspiration for myocardial infarction. N Engl J Med, 2014, 371 (12): 1111-1120.

[159] Jolly SS, Cairns JA, Yusuf S, et al. Randomized trial of primary PCI with or without routine manual thrombectomy. N Engl J Med, 2015, 372 (15): 1389-1398.

[160] Jolly SS, Cairns JA, Yusuf S, et al. Outcomes after thrombus aspiration for ST elevation myocardial infarction: 1-year follow-up of the prospective randomised TOTAL trial. Lancet, 2016, 387 (10014): 127-135.

[161] Jolly SS, Cairns JA, Yusuf S, et al. Stroke in the TOTAL trial: a randomized trial of routine thrombectomy vs. percutaneous coronary intervention alone in ST elevation myocardial

infarction. Eur Heart J, 2015, 36 (35): 2364-2372.

[162] Jolly SS, James S, Dzavik V, et al. Thrombus aspiration in ST-segment-elevation myocardial infarction. An individual patient meta-analysis: Thrombectomy Trialists Collaboration. Circulation, 2017, 135 (2): 143-152.

[163] Sorajja P, Gersh BJ, Cox DA, et al. Impact of multivessel disease on reperfusion success and clinical outcomes in patients undergoing primary percutaneous coronary intervention for acute myocardial infarction. Eur Heart J, 2007, 28 (14): 1709-1716.

[164] Dziewierz A, Siudak Z, Rakowski T, et al. Impact of multivessel coronary artery disease and noninfarct-related artery revascularization on outcome of patients with ST-elevation myocardial infarction transferred for primary percutaneous coronary intervention (from the EUROTRANSFER Registry). Am J Cardiol, 2010, 106 (3): 342-347.

[165] Cavender MA, Milford-Beland S, Roe MT, et al. Prevalence, predictors, and in-hospital outcomes of non-infarct artery intervention during primary percutaneous coronary intervention for ST-segment elevation myocardial infarction (from the National Cardiovascular Data Registry). Am J Cardiol, 2009, 104 (4): 507-513.

[166] Hannan EL, Samadashvili Z, Walford G, et al. Culprit vessel percutaneous coronary intervention versus multivessel and staged percutaneous coronary intervention for ST-segment elevation myocardial infarction patients with multivessel disease. JACC Cardiovasc Interv, 2010, 3 (1): 22-31.

[167] Politi L, Sgura F, Rossi R, et al. A randomised trial of target-vessel versus multi-vessel revascularisation in ST-elevation myocardial infarction: major adverse cardiac events during long-term follow-up. Heart, 2010, 96 (9): 662-667.

[168] Wald DS, Morris JK, Wald NJ, et al. Randomized trial of preventive angioplasty in myocardial infarction. N Engl J Med, 2013, 369 (12): 1115-1123.

[169] Gershlick AH, Khan JN, Kelly DJ, et al. Randomized trial of complete versus lesion-only revascularization in patients undergoing primary percutaneous coronary intervention for STEMI and multivessel disease: the CvLPRIT trial. J Am Coll Cardiol, 2015, 65 (10): 963-972.

[170] Engstrom T, Kelbaek H, Helqvist S, et al. Complete revascularisation versus treatment of the culprit lesion only in patients with ST-segment elevation myocardial infarction and

multivessel disease (DANAMI-3-PRIMULTI): an open-label, randomised controlled trial. Lancet, 2015, 386 (9994): 665-671.

[171] Smits PC, Abdel-Wahab M, Neumann FJ, et al. Fractional flow reserve-guided multivessel angioplasty in myocardial infarction. N Engl J Med, 2017, 376 (13): 1234-1244.

[172] Moreno R, Mehta SR. Nonculprit vessel intervention: let's COMPLETE the evidence. Rev Esp Cardiol (English Ed) , 2017, 70: 418-420.

[173] Bangalore S, Toklu B, Wetterslev J. Complete versus culprit-only revascularization for ST-segment-elevation myocardial infarction and multivessel disease: a meta-analysis and trial sequential analysis of randomized trials. Circ Cardiovasc Interv, 2015, 8 (4): e002142.

[174] Elgendy IY, Mahmoud AN, Kumbhani DJ, et al. Complete or culprit-only revascularization for patients with multivessel coronary artery disease undergoing percutaneous coronary intervention: a pairwise and network meta-analysis of randomized trials. JACC Cardiovasc Interv, 2017, 10 (4): 315-324.

[175] Patel MR, Smalling RW, Thiele H, et al. Intra-aortic balloon counterpulsation and infarct size in patients with acute anterior myocardial infarction without shock: the CRISP AMI randomized trial. JAMA, 2011, 306 (12): 1329-1337.

[176] Sjauw KD, Engstrom AE, Vis MM, et al. A systematic review and Metaanalysis of intra-aortic balloon pump therapy in ST-elevation myocardial infarction: should we change the guidelines?Eur Heart J, 2009, 30 (4): 459-468.

[177] Thiele H, Zeymer U, Neumann FJ, et al. Intraaortic balloon support for myocardial infarction with cardiogenic shock. N Engl J Med, 2012, 367 (14): 1287-1296.

[178] Stefanini GG, Byrne RA, Serruys PW, et al. Biodegradable polymer drug-eluting stents reduce the risk of stent thrombosis at 4 years in patients undergoing percutaneous coronary intervention: a pooled analysis of individual patient data from the ISAR-TEST 3, ISAR-TEST 4, and LEADERS randomized trials. Eur Heart J, 2012, 33 (10): 1214-1222.

[179] Palmerini T, Biondi-Zoccai G, Della Riva D, et al. Clinical outcomes with drug-eluting and bare-Metal stents in patients with ST-segment elevation myocardial infarction: evidence from a comprehensive network meta-analysis. J Am Coll Cardiol, 2013, 62 (6): 496-504.

[180] Karrowni W, Vyas A, Giacomino B, et al. Radial versus femoral access for primary percutaneous interventions in STsegment elevation myocardial infarction patients: a meta-

analysis of randomized controlled trials. JACC Cardiovasc Interv, 2013, 6 (8): 814-823.

[181]   Zeymer U, Hohlfeld T, Vom Dahl J, et al. Prospective, randomised trial of the time dependent antiplatelet effects of 500 mg and 250 mg acetylsalicylic acid i. v. and 300 mg p. o. in ACS (ACUTE). Thromb Haemost, 2017, 117 (3): 625-635.

[182]   Montalescot G, van 't Hof AW, Lapostolle F, et al. Prehospital ticagrelor in ST-segment elevation myocardial infarction. N Engl J Med, 2014, 371 (11): 1016-1027.

[183]   Koul S, Smith JG, Schersten F, et al. Effect of upstream clopidogrel treatment in patients with ST-segment elevation myocardial infarction undergoing primary percutaneous coronary intervention. Eur Heart J, 2011, 32 (23): 2989-2997.

[184]   Dorler J, Edlinger M, Alber HF, et al. Clopidogrel pre-treatment is associated with reduced in-hospital mortality in primary percutaneous coronary intervention for acute ST-elevation myocardial infarction. Eur Heart J, 2011, 32 (23): 2954-2961.

[185]   Zeymer U, Arntz HR, Mark B, et al. Efficacy and safety of a high loading dose of clopidogrel administered prehospitally to improve primary percutaneous coronary intervention in acute myocardial infarction: the randomized CIPAMI trial. Clin Res Cardiol, 2012, 101 (4): 305-312.

[186]   Wiviott SD, Braunwald E, McCabe CH, et al. Prasugrel versus clopidogrel in patients with acute coronary syndromes. N Engl J Med, 2007, 357 (20): 2001-2015.

[187]   Wallentin L, Becker RC, Budaj A, et al. Ticagrelor versus clopidogrel in patients with acute coronary syndromes. N Engl J Med, 2009, 361 (11): 1045-1057.

[188]   Roe MT, Armstrong PW, Fox KA, et al. Prasugrel versus clopidogrel for acute coronary syndromes without revascularization. N Engl J Med, 2012, 367 (14): 1297-1309.

[189]   Storey RF, Becker RC, Harrington RA, et al. Characterization of dyspnoea in PLATO study patients treated with ticagrelor or clopidogrel and its association with clinical outcomes. Eur Heart J, 2011, 32 (23): 2945-2953.

[190]   Mehta SR, Tanguay JF, Eikelboom JW, et al. Double-dose versus standard-dose clopidogrel and high-dose versus low-dose aspirin in individuals undergoing percutaneous coronary intervention for acute coronary syndromes (CURRENT-OASIS 7): a randomised factorial trial. Lancet, 2010, 376 (9748): 1233-1243.

[191]   Bhatt DL, Lincoff AM, Gibson CM, et al. Intravenous platelet blockade with cangrelor during

PCI. N Engl J Med, 2009, 361 (24): 2330-2341.

[192] Harrington RA, Stone GW, McNulty S, et al. Platelet inhibition with cangrelor in patients undergoing PCI. N Engl J Med, 2009, 361 (24): 2318-2329.

[193] Bhatt DL, Stone GW, Mahaffey KW, et al. Effect of platelet inhibition with cangrelor during PCI on ischemic events. N Engl J Med, 2013, 368 (14): 1303-1313.

[194] Steg PG, Bhatt DL, Hamm CW, et al. Effect of cangrelor on periprocedural outcomes in percutaneous coronary interventions: a pooled analysis of patient-level data. Lancet, 2013, 382 (9909): 1981-1992.

[195] Ellis SG, Tendera M, de Belder MA, et al. Facilitated PCI in patients with ST-elevation myocardial infarction. N Engl J Med, 2008, 358 (21): 2205-2217.

[196] ten Berg JM, van 't Hof AW, Dill T, et al. Effect of early, pre-hospital initiation of high bolus dose tirofiban in patients with ST segment elevation myocardial infarction on short- and long-term clinical outcome. J Am Coll Cardiol, 2010, 55 (22): 2446-2455.

[197] Stone GW, Witzenbichler B, Guagliumi G, et al. Bivalirudin during primary PCI in acute myocardial infarction. N Engl J Med, 2008, 358 (21): 2218-2230.

[198] Friedland S, Eisenberg MJ, Shimony A. Meta-analysis of randomized controlled trials of intracoronary versus intravenous administration of glycoprotein II b/ III a inhibitors during percutaneous coronary intervention for acute coronary syndrome. Am J Cardiol, 2011, 108 (9): 1244-1251.

[199] Yusuf S, Mehta SR, Chrolavicius S, Afzal R, et al. Effects of fondaparinux on mortality and reinfarction in patients with acute STsegment elevation myocardial infarction: the OASIS-6 randomized trial. JAMA, 2006, 295 (13): 1519-1530.

[200] Montalescot G, Zeymer U, Silvain J, et al. Intravenous enoxaparin or unfractionated heparin in primary percutaneous coronary intervention for STelevation myocardial infarction: the international randomised open-label ATOLL trial. Lancet, 2011, 378 (9792): 693-703.

[201] Collet JP, Huber K, Cohen M, et al. A direct comparison of intravenous enoxaparin with unfractionated heparin in primary percutaneous coronary intervention (from the ATOLL trial). Am J Cardiol, 2013, 112 (9): 1367-1372.

[202] Silvain J, Beygui F, Barthelemy O, et al. Efficacy and safety of enoxaparin versus unfractionated heparin during percutaneous coronary intervention: systematic review and

meta-analysis. BMJ, 2012, 344: e553.

[203] Steg PG, van't Hof A, Hamm CW, et al. Bivalirudin started during emergency transport for primary PCI. N Engl J Med, 2013, 369 (23): 2207-2217.

[204] Schulz S, Richardt G, Laugwitz KL, et al. Prasugrel plus bivalirudin vs. clopidogrel plus heparin in patients with ST-segment elevation myocardial infarction. Eur Heart J, 2014, 35 (34): 2285-2294.

[205] Shahzad A, Kemp I, Mars C, et al. Unfractionated heparin versus bivalirudin in primary percutaneous coronary intervention (HEAT-PPCI): an open-label, single centre, randomised controlled trial. Lancet, 2014, 384 (9957): 1849-1858.

[206] Han Y, Guo J, Zheng Y, et al. Bivalirudin vs heparin with or without tirofiban during primary percutaneous coronary intervention in acute myocardial infarction: the BRIGHT randomized clinical trial. JAMA, 2015, 313 (13): 1336-1346.

[207] Zeymer U, van 't Hof A, Adgey J, et al. Bivalirudin is superior to heparins alone with bailout GP IIb/IIIa inhibitors in patients with ST-segment elevation myocardial infarction transported emergently for primary percutaneous coronary intervention: a pre-specified analysis from the EUROMAX trial. Eur Heart J, 2014, 35 (36): 2460-2467.

[208] Capodanno D, Gargiulo G, Capranzano P, et al. Bivalirudin versus heparin with or without glycoprotein Ⅱ b/ Ⅲ a inhibitors in patients with STEMI undergoing primary PCI: An updated meta-analysis of 10350 patients from five randomized clinical trials. Eur Heart J Acute Cardiovasc Care, 2016, 5 (3): 253-262.

[209] Valgimigli M, Frigoli E, Leonardi S, et al. Bivalirudin or unfractionated heparin in acute coronary syndromes. N Engl J Med, 2015, 373 (11): 997-1009.

[210] Leonardi S, Frigoli E, Rothenbuhler M, et al. Bivalirudin or unfractionated heparin in patients with acute coronary syndromes managed invasively with and without ST elevation (MATRIX): randomised controlled trial. BMJ, 2016, 354: i4935.

[211] Kastrati A, Neumann FJ, Mehilli J, et al. Bivalirudin versus unfractionated heparin during percutaneous coronary intervention. N Engl J Med, 2008, 359 (7): 688-696.

[212] Ndrepepa G, Schulz S, Keta D, et al. Bleeding after percutaneous coronary intervention with Bivalirudin or unfractionated Heparin and one-year mortality. Am J Cardiol, 2010, 105 (2): 163-167.

[213] ISIS-2 (Second International Study of Infarct Survival) Collaborative Group. Randomised trial of intravenous streptokinase, oral aspirin, both, or neither among 17187 cases of suspected acute myocardial infarction: ISIS-2. Lancet, 1988, 2 (8607): 349-360.

[214] Patrono C, Andreotti F, Arnesen H, et al. Antiplatelet agents for the treatment and prevention of atherothrombosis. Eur Heart J, 2011, 32 (23): 2922-2932.

[215] Cavender MA, Sabatine MS. Bivalirudin versus heparin in patients planned for percutaneous coronary intervention: a meta-analysis of randomised controlled trials. Lancet, 2014, 384 (9943): 599-606.

[216] Stone GW, Selker HP, Thiele H, et al. Relationship between infarct size and outcomes following primary PCI: patient-level analysis from 10 randomized trials. J Am Coll Cardiol, 2016, 67 (14): 1674-1683.

[217] Ibanez B, Heusch G, Ovize M, et al Evolving therapies for myocardial ischemia/reperfusion injury. J Am Coll Cardiol, 2015, 65 (14): 1454-1471.

[218] Niccoli G, Scalone G, Lerman A, et al. Coronary microvascular obstruction in acute myocardial infarction. Eur Heart J, 2016, 37 (13): 1024-1033.

[219] Hausenloy DJ, Botker HE, Engstrom T, et al. Targeting reperfusion injury in patients with ST-segment elevation myocardial infarction: trials and tribulations. Eur Heart J, 2017, 38 (13): 935-941.

[220] Fibrinolytic Therapy Trialists' (FTT) Collaborative Group. Indications for fibrinolytic therapy in suspected acute myocardial infarction: collaborative overview of early mortality and major morbidity results from all randomised trials of more than 1000 patients. Lancet, 1994, 343 (8893): 311-322.

[221] White HD. Thrombolytic therapy in the elderly. Lancet, 2000, 356 (9247): 2028-2030.

[222] Bonnefoy E, Lapostolle F, Leizorovicz A, et al. Primary angioplasty versus prehospital fibrinolysis in acute myocardial infarction: a randomised study. Lancet, 2002, 360 (9336): 825-829.

[223] Assessment of the Safety and Efficacy of a New Thrombolytic (ASSENT-2) Investigators, Van de Werf F, Adgey J, et al. Single-bolus tenecteplase compared with front-loaded alteplase in acute myocardial infarction: the ASSENT-2 doubleblind randomised trial. Lancet, 1999, 354 (9180): 716-722.

[224] GUSTO Investigators. An international randomized trial comparing four thrombolytic strategies for acute myocardial infarction. N Engl J Med, 1993, 329 (10): 673-682.

[225] Chen ZM, Jiang LX, Chen YP, et al. Addition of clopidogrel to aspirin in 45852 patients with acute myocardial infarction: randomised placebo-controlled trial. Lancet, 2005, 366 (9497): 1607-1621.

[226] Sabatine MS, Cannon CP, Gibson CM, et al. Addition of clopidogrel to aspirin and fibrinolytic therapy for myocardial infarction with ST-segment elevation. N Engl J Med, 2005, 352 (12): 1179-1189.

[227] Assessment of the Safety and Efficacy of a New Thrombolytic Regimen (ASSENT) -3 Investigators. Efficacy and safety of tenecteplase in combination with enoxaparin, abciximab, or unfractionated heparin: the ASSENT-3 randomised trial in acute myocardial infarction. Lancet, 2001, 358 (9282): 605-613.

[228] Wallentin L, Goldstein P, Armstrong PW, et al. Efficacy and safety of tenecteplase in combination with the low-molecularweight heparin enoxaparin or unfractionated heparin in the prehospital setting: the Assessment of the Safety and Efficacy of a New Thrombolytic Regimen (ASSENT) -3 PLUS randomized trial in acute myocardial infarction. Circulation, 2003, 108 (2): 135-142.

[229] Giraldez RR, Nicolau JC, Corbalan R, et al. Enoxaparin is superior to unfractionated heparin in patients with ST elevation myocardial infarction undergoing fibrinolysis regardless of the choice of lytic: an ExTRACT-TIMI 25 analysis. Eur Heart J, 2007, 28 (13): 1566-1573.

[230] White HD, Braunwald E, Murphy SA, et al. Enoxaparin vs. unfractionated heparin with fibrinolysis for STelevation myocardial infarction in elderly and younger patients: results from ExTRACT-TIMI 25. Eur Heart J, 2007, 28 (9): 1066-1071.

[231] Ross AM, Molhoek P, Lundergan C, et al. Randomized comparison of enoxaparin, a low-molecular-weight heparin, with unfractionated heparin adjunctive to recombinant tissue plasminogen activator thrombolysis and aspirin: second trial of Heparin and Aspirin Reperfusion Therapy (HART II). Circulation, 2001, 104 (6): 648-652.

[232] Antman EM, Louwerenburg HW, Baars HF, et al. Enoxaparin as adjunctive antithrombin therapy for ST-elevation myocardial infarction: results of the ENTIRE-Thrombolysis in Myocardial Infarction (TIMI) 23 Trial. Circulation, 2002, 105 (14): 1642-1649.

[233] Peters RJ, Joyner C, Bassand JP, et al. The role of fondaparinux as an adjunct to thrombolytic therapy in acute myocardial infarction: a subgroup analysis of the OASIS-6 trial. Eur Heart J, 2008, 29 (3): 324-331.

[234] Fernandez-Aviles F, Alonso JJ, Castro-Beiras A, et al. Routine invasive strategy within 24 hours of thrombolysis versus ischaemia-guided conservative approach for acute myocardial infarction with ST-segment elevation (GRACIA-1): a randomised controlled trial. Lancet, 2004, 364 (9439): 1045-1053.

[235] Hochman JS, Sleeper LA, White HD, et al. One-year survival following early revascularization for cardiogenic shock. JAMA, 2001, 285 (2): 190-192.

[236] Ellis SG, da Silva ER, Heyndrickx G, et al. Randomized comparison of rescue angioplasty with conservative management of patients with early failure of thrombolysis for acute anterior myocardial infarction. Circulation, 1994, 90 (5): 2280-2284.

[237] Assessment of the Safety and Efficacy of a New Treatment Strategy with Percutaneous Coronary Intervention (ASSENT-4 PCI) Investigators. Primary versus tenecteplase-facilitated percutaneous coronary intervention in patients with ST-segment elevation acute myocardial infarction (ASSENT-4 PCI): randomised trial. Lancet, 2006, 367 (9510): 569-578.

[238] Sinnaeve PR, Armstrong PW, Gershlick AH, et al. ST-segment-elevation myocardial infarction patients randomized to a pharmaco-invasive strategy or primary percutaneous coronary intervention: Strategic Reperfusion Early After Myocardial Infarction (STREAM) 1-year mortality follow-up. Circulation, 2014, 130 (14): 1139-1145.

[239] Scheller B, Hennen B, Hammer B, et al. Beneficial effects of immediate stenting after thrombolysis in acute myocardial infarction. J Am Coll Cardiol, 2003, 42 (4): 634-641.

[240] Le May MR, Wells GA, Labinaz M, et al. Combined angioplasty and pharmacological intervention versus thrombolysis alone in acute myocardial infarction (CAPITAL AMI study). J Am Coll Cardiol, 2005, 46 (3): 417-424.

[241] Abdel-Qadir H, Yan AT, Tan M, et al. Consistency of benefit from an early invasive strategy after fibrinolysis: a patient-level meta-analysis. Heart, 2015, 101 (19): 1554-1561.

[242] Sanchez PL, Gimeno F, Ancillo P, et al. Role of the paclitaxel-eluting stent and tirofiban in patients with ST-elevation myocardial infarction undergoing postfibrinolysis angioplasty: the GRACIA-3 randomized clinical trial. Circ Cardiovasc Interv, 2010, 3 (4): 297-307.

[243] White HD, Hirulog and Early Reperfusion or Occlusion (HERO) -2 Trial Investigators. Thrombin-specific anticoagulation with bivalirudin versus heparin in patients receiving fibrinolytic therapy for acute myocardial infarction: the HERO-2 randomised trial. Lancet, 2001, 358 (9296): 1855-1863.

[244] Fernandez-Aviles F, Alonso JJ, Pena G, et al. Primary angioplasty vs. early routine postfibrinolysis angioplasty for acute myocardial infarction with ST-segment elevation: the GRACIA-2 non-inferiority, randomized, controlled trial. Eur Heart J, 2007, 28 (8): 949-960.

[245] Van de Werf F, Barron HV, Armstrong PW, et al. Incidence and predictors of bleeding events after fibrinolytic therapy with fibrin-specific agents: a comparison of TNK-tPA and rt-PA. Eur Heart J, 2001, 22 (24): 2253-2261.

[246] Global Use of Strategies to Open Occluded Coronary Arteries (GUSTO III) Investigators. A comparison of reteplase with alteplase for acute myocardial infarction. N Engl J Med, 1997, 337 (16): 1118-1123.

[247] Bottiger BW, Arntz HR, Chamberlain DA, et al. Thrombolysis during resuscitation for outof-hospital cardiac arrest. N Engl J Med, 2008, 359 (25): 2651-2662.

[248] Hochman JS, Sleeper LA, Webb JG, et al. Early revascularization in acute myocardial infarction complicated by cardiogenic shock. SHOCK Investigators. Should We Emergently Revascularize Occluded Coronaries for Cardiogenic Shock. N Engl J Med, 1999, 341 (9): 625-634.

[249] Weiss ES, Chang DD, Joyce DL, et al. Optimal timing of coronary artery bypass after acute myocardial infarction: a review of California discharge data. J Thorac Cardiovasc Surg, 2008, 135 (3): 503-511.

[250] Hansson EC, Jideus L, Aberg B, et al. Coronary artery bypass grafting-related bleeding complications in patients treated with ticagrelor or clopidogrel: a nationwide study. Eur Heart J, 2016, 37 (2): 189-197.

[251] Deja MA, Kargul T, Domaradzki W, et al. Effects of preoperative aspirin in coronary artery bypass grafting: a double-blind, placebo-controlled, randomized trial. J Thorac Cardiovasc Surg, 2012, 144 (1): 204-209.

[252] Lim E, Ali Z, Ali A, et al. Indirect comparison meta-analysis of aspirin therapy after coronary surgery. BMJ, 2003, 327 (7427): 1309.

[253] Gavaghan TP, Gebski V, Baron DW. Immediate postoperative aspirin improves vein graft patency early and late after coronary artery bypass graft surgery. A placebo-controlled, randomized study. Circulation, 1991, 83 (5): 1526-1533.

[254] Hasin Y, Danchin N, Filippatos GS, et al. Recommendations for the structure, organization, and operation of intensive cardiac care units. Eur Heart J, 2005, 26 (16): 1676-1682.

[255] Spencer FA, Lessard D, Gore JM, et al. Declining length of hospital stay for acute myocardial infarction and postdischarge outcomes: a community-wide perspective. Arch Intern Med, 2004, 164 (7): 733-740.

[256] Berger AK, Duval S, Jacobs DR, et al. Relation of length of hospital stay in acute myocardial infarction to postdischarge mortality. Am J Cardiol, 2008, 101 (4): 428-434.

[257] Grines CL, Marsalese DL, Brodie B, et al. Safety and cost-effectiveness of early discharge after primary angioplasty in low risk patients with acute myocardial infarction. PAMI- II Investigators. Primary Angioplasty in Myocardial Infarction. J Am Coll Cardiol, 1998, 31 (5): 967-972.

[258] De Luca G, Suryapranata H, van't Hof AW, et al. Prognostic assessment of patients with acute myocardial infarction treated with primary angioplasty: implications for early discharge. Circulation, 2004, 109 (22): 2737-2743.

[259] Azzalini L, Sole E, Sans J, et al. Feasibility and safety of an early discharge strategy after low-risk acute myocardial infarction treated with primary percutaneous coronary intervention: the EDAMI pilot trial. Cardiology, 2015, 130 (2): 120-129.

[260] Melberg T, Jorgensen M, Orn S, et al. Safety and health status following early discharge in patients with acute myocardial infarction treated with primary PCI: a randomized trial. Eur J Prev Cardiol, 2015, 22 (11): 1427-1434.

[261] Noman A, Zaman AG, Schechter C, et al. Early discharge after primary percutaneous coronary intervention for ST-elevation myocardial infarction. Eur Heart J Acute Cardiovasc Care, 2013, 2 (3): 262-269.

[262] Jones DA, Rathod KS, Howard JP, et al. Safety and feasibility of hospital discharge 2 days following primary percutaneous intervention for ST-segment elevation myocardial infarction. Heart, 2012, 98 (23): 1722-1727.

[263] Estévez-Loureiro R, Calviño-Santos R, Vázquez JM, et al. Safety and feasibility of returning

patients early to their originating centers after transfer for primary percutaneous coronary intervention. Rev Esp Cardiol, 2009, 62 (12): 1356-1364.

[264] Morrow DA, Antman EM, Charlesworth A, et al. TIMI risk score for ST-elevation myocardial infarction: A convenient, bedside, clinical score for risk assessment at presentation: An intravenous nPA for treatment of infarcting myocardium early II trial substudy. Circulation, 2000, 102 (17): 2031-2037.

[265] Newby LK, Hasselblad V, Armstrong PW, et al. Time-based risk assessment after myocardial infarction. Implications for timing of discharge and applications to medical decision-making. Eur Heart J, 2003, 24 (2): 182-189.

[266] Dans AL, Connolly SJ, Wallentin L, et al. Concomitant use of antiplatelet therapy with dabigatran or warfarin in the Randomized Evaluation of Long-Term Anticoagulation Therapy (RE-LY) trial. Circulation, 2013, 127 (5): 634-640.

[267] Sørensen R, Hansen ML, Abildstrom SZ, et al. Risk of bleeding in patients with acute myocardial infarction treated with different combinations of aspirin, clopidogrel, and vitamin K antagonists in Denmark: a retrospective analysis of nationwide registry data. Lancet, 2009, 374 (9706): 1967-1974.

[268] Hansen ML, Sørensen R, Clausen MT, et al. Risk of bleeding with single, dual, or triple therapy with warfarin, aspirin, and clopidogrel in patients with atrial fibrillation. Arch Intern Med, 2010, 170 (16): 1433-1441.

[269] Oldgren J, Budaj A, Granger CB, et al. Dabigatran vs. placebo in patients with acute coronary syndromes on dual antiplatelet therapy: a randomized, double-blind, phase II trial. Eur Heart J, 2011, 32 (22): 2781-2789.

[270] Barnes GD, Gu X, Haymart B, et al. The predictive ability of the CHADS2 and CHA2DS2-VASc scores for bleeding risk in atrial fibrillation: the MAQI (2) experience. Thromb Res, 2014, 134 (2): 294-299.

[271] Roldán V, Marín F, Manzano-Fernández S, et al. The HAS-BLED score has better prediction accuracy for major bleeding than CHADS2 or CHA2DS2-VASc scores in anticoagulated patients with atrial fibrillation. J Am Coll Cardiol, 2013, 62 (23): 2199-2204.

[272] Gibson CM, Mehran R, Bode C, et al. Prevention of bleeding in patients with atrial fibrillation undergoing PCI. N Engl J Med, 2016, 375 (25): 2423-2434.

[273] Toleva O, Ibrahim Q, Brass N, et al. Treatment choices in elderly patients with ST: elevation myocardial infarction-insights from the Vital Heart Response registry. Open Heart, 2015, 2 (1): e000235.

[274] Malkin CJ, Prakash R, Chew DP. The impact of increased age on outcome from a strategy of early invasive management and revascularisation in patients with acute coronary syndromes: retrospective analysis study from the ACACIA registry. BMJ Open, 2012, 2 (1): e000540.

[275] Alexander KP, Chen AY, Roe MT, et al. Excess dosing of antiplatelet and antithrombin agents in the treatment of non- ST-segment elevation acute coronary syndromes. JAMA, 2005, 294 (24): 3108-3116.

[276] Bueno H, Betriu A, Heras M, et al. Primary angioplasty vs. fibrinolysis in very old patients with acute myocardial infarction: TRIANA (TRatamiento del Infarto Agudo de miocardio eN Ancianos) randomized trial and pooled analysis with previous studies. Eur Heart J, 2011, 32 (1): 51-60.

[277] Szummer K, Lundman P, Jacobson SH, et al. Relation between renal function, presentation, use of therapies and in-hospital complications in acute coronary syndrome: data from the SWEDEHEART register. J Intern Med, 2010, 268 (1): 40-49.

[278] Timmer JR, Ottervanger JP, de Boer MJ, et al. Primary percutaneous coronary intervention compared with fibrinolysis for myocardial infarction in diabetes mellitus: results from the Primary Coronary Angioplasty vs Thrombolysis-2 trial. Arch Intern Med, 2007, 167 (13): 1353-1359.

[279] Alderman EL, Kip KE, Whitlow PL, et al. Native coronary disease progression exceeds failed revascularization as cause of angina after five years in the Bypass Angioplasty Revascularization Investigation (BARI). J Am Coll Cardiol, 2004, 44 (4): 766-774.

[280] James S, Angiolillo DJ, Cornel JH, et al. Ticagrelor vs. clopidogrel in patients with acute coronary syndromes and diabetes: a substudy from the PLATelet inhibition and patient Outcomes (PLATO) trial. Eur Heart J, 2010, 31 (24): 3006-3016.

[281] NICE-SUGAR Study Investigators, Finfer S, Chittock DR, et al. Intensive versus conventional glucose control in critically ill patients. N Engl J Med, 2009, 360 (13): 1283-1297.

[282] Senthinathan A, Kelly V, Dzingina M, et al. Hyperglycaemia in acute coronary syndromes:

summary of NICE guidance. BMJ, 2011, 343: d6646.

[283] Fox KA, Dabbous OH, Goldberg RJ, et al. Prediction of risk of death and myocardial infarction in the six months after presentation with acute coronary syndrome: prospective multinational observational study (GRACE). BMJ, 2006, 333 (7578): 1091.

[284] Fox KA, Fitzgerald G, Puymirat E, et al. Should patients with acute coronary disease be stratified for management according to their risk?Derivation, external validation and outcomes using the updated GRACE risk score. BMJ Open, 2014, 4 (2): e004425.

[285] van Loon RB, Veen G, Baur LH, et al. Improved clinical outcome after invasive management of patients with recent myocardial infarction and proven myocardial viability: primary results of a randomized controlled trial (VIAMI-trial). Trials, 2012, 13: 1.

[286] van Loon RB, Veen G, Baur LH, et al. Long-term follow-up of the viability guided angioplasty after acute myocardial infarction (VIAMI) trial. Int J Cardiol, 2015, 186: 111-116.

[287] Nesković AN, Bojić M, Popović AD. Detection of significant residual stenosis of the infarct-related artery after thrombolysis by high-dose dipyridamole echocardiography test: is it detected often enough?Clin Cardiol, 1997, 20 (6): 569-572.

[288] Kim RJ, Wu E, Rafael A, et al. The use of contrast-enhanced magnetic resonance imaging to identify reversible myocardial dysfunction. N Engl J Med, 2000, 343 (20): 1445-1453.

[289] La Canna G, Rahimtoola SH, Visioli O, et al. Sensitivity, specificity, and predictive accuracies of non-invasive tests, singly and in combination, for diagnosis of hibernating myocardium. Eur Heart J, 2000, 21 (16): 1358-1367.

[290] Gerber BL, Rousseau MF, Ahn SA, et al. Prognostic value of myocardial viability by delayed-enhanced magnetic resonance in patients with coronary artery disease and low ejection fraction: impact of revascularization therapy. J Am Coll Cardiol, 2012, 59 (9): 825-835.

[291] Shah DJ, Kim HW, James O, et al. Prevalence of regional myocardial thinning and relationship with myocardial scarring in patients with coronary artery disease. JAMA, 2013, 309 (9): 909-918.

[292] Beanlands RS, Nichol G, Huszti E, et al. F-18-fluorodeoxyglucose positron emission tomography imaging-assisted management of patients with severe left ventricular dysfunction and suspected coronary disease: a randomized, controlled trial (PARR- 2). J Am Coll Cardiol,

2007, 50 (20): 2002-2012.

[293] Allman KC, Shaw LJ, Hachamovitch R, et al. Myocardial viability testing and impact of revascularization on prognosis in patients with coronary artery disease and left ventricular dysfunction: a meta-analysis. J Am Coll Cardiol, 2002, 39 (7): 1151-1158.

[294] Eitel I, de Waha S, Wöhrle J, et al. Comprehensive prognosis assessment by CMR imaging after ST-segment elevation myocardial infarction. J Am Coll Cardiol, 2014, 64 (12): 1217-1226.

[295] Neskovic AN, Hagendorff A, Lancellotti P, et al. Emergency echocardiography: the European Association of Cardiovascular Imaging recommendations. Eur Heart J Cardiovasc Imaging, 2013, 14 (1): 1-11.

[296] Søholm H, Lønborg J, Andersen MJ, et al. Repeated echocardiography after first ever ST-segment elevation myocardial infarction treated with primary percutaneous coronary intervention—is it necessary?Eur Heart J Acute Cardiovasc Care, 2015, 4 (6): 528-536.

[297] St John Sutton M, Pfeffer MA, Plappert T, et al. Quantitative two-dimensional echocardiographic measurements are major predictors of adverse cardiovascular events after acute myocardial infarction. The protective effects of captopril. Circulation, 1994, 89 (1): 68-75.

[298] Carlos ME, Smart SC, Wynsen JC, et al. Dobutamine stress echocardiography for risk stratification after myocardial infarction. Circulation, 1997, 95 (6): 1402-1410.

[299] Brown KA, Heller GV, Landin RS, et al. Early dipyridamole (99m) Tc-sestamibi single photon emission computed tomographic imaging 2 to 4 days after acute myocardial infarction predicts in-hospital and postdischarge cardiac events: comparison with submaximal exercise imaging. Circulation, 1999, 100 (20): 2060-2066.

[300] Bulluck H, White SK, Fröhlich GM, et al. Quantifying the area at risk in reperfused ST-Segment-Elevation myocardial infarction patients using hybrid cardiac positron emission tomography-magnetic resonance imaging. Circ Cardiovasc Imaging, 2016, 9 (3): e003900.

[301] Chow CK, Jolly S, Rao-Melacini P, et al. Association of diet, exercise, and smoking modification with risk of early cardiovascular events after acute coronary syndromes. Circulation, 2010, 121 (6): 750-758.

[302] Thomson CC, Rigotti NA. Hospital- and clinic-based smoking cessation interventions for

smokers with cardiovascular disease. Prog Cardiovasc Dis, 2003, 45 (6): 459-479.

[303] Rigotti NA, Clair C, Munafò MR, et al. Interventions for smoking cessation in hospitalised patients. Cochrane Database Syst Rev, 2012, 5: CD001837.

[304] Critchley JA, Capewell S. Mortality risk reduction associated with smoking cessation in patients with coronary heart disease: a systematic review. JAMA, 2003, 290 (1): 86-97.

[305] Rallidis LS, Pavlakis G. The fundamental importance of smoking cessation in those with premature ST-segment elevation acute myocardial infarction. Curr Opin Cardiol, 2016, 31 (5): 531-536.

[306] Stead LF, Koilpillai P, Fanshawe TR, et al. Combined pharmacotherapy and behavioural interventions for smoking cessation. Cochrane Database Syst Rev, 2016, 3: CD008286.

[307] McRobbie H, Bullen C, Hartmann-Boyce J, et al. Electronic cigarettes for smoking cessation and reduction. Cochrane Database Syst Rev, 2014, 12(12): CD010216.

[308] Global BMI Mortality Collaboration, Di Angelantonio E, Bhupathiraju ShN, et al. Body-mass index and all-cause mortality: individualparticipant- data meta-analysis of 239 prospective studies in four continents. Lancet, 2016, 388 (10046): 776-786.

[309] Anderson L, Oldridge N, Thompson DR, et al. Exercise-based cardiac rehabilitation for coronary heart disease: cochrane systematic review and meta-analysis. J Am Coll Cardiol, 2016, 67 (1): 1-12.

[310] Taylor RS, Brown A, Ebrahim S, et al. Exercise-based rehabilitation for patients with coronary heart disease: systematic review and meta-analysis of randomized controlled trials. Am J Med, 2004, 116 (10): 682-692.

[311] Dalal HM, Zawada A, Jolly K, et al. Home based versus centre based cardiac rehabilitation: cochrane systematic review and meta-analysis. BMJ, 2010, 340: b5631.

[312] European Association of Cardiovascular Prevention and Rehabilitation Committee for Science Guidelines, EACPR, Corrà U, et al. Secondary prevention through cardiac rehabilitation: physical activity counselling and exercise training: key components of the position paper from the Cardiac Rehabilitation Section of the European Association of Cardiovascular Prevention and Rehabilitation. Eur Heart J, 2010, 31 (16): 1967-1974.

[313] Dreyer RP, Xu X, Zhang W, et al. Return to work after acute myocardial infarction: comparison between young women and men. Circ Cardiovasc Qual Outcomes, 2016, 9 (2

Suppl 1): S45-S52.

[314] Smith D, Toff W, Joy M, et al. Fitness to fly for passengers with cardiovascular disease. Heart, 2010, 96 (Suppl 2): ii1–ii16.

[315] SPRINT Research Group, Wright JT Jr, Williamson JD, et al. A randomized trial of intensive versus standard blood-pressure control. N Engl J Med, 2015, 373 (22): 2103-2116.

[316] Lonn EM, Bosch J, López-Jaramillo P, et al. Blood-pressure lowering in intermediate-risk persons without cardiovascular disease. N Engl J Med, 2016, 374 (21): 2009-2020.

[317] Simpson SH, Eurich DT, Majumdar SR, et al. A meta-analysis of the association between adherence to drug therapy and mortality. BMJ, 2006, 333 (7557): 15.

[318] Faridi KF, Peterson ED, McCoy LA, et al. Timing of first postdischarge follow-up and medication adherence after acute myocardial infarction. JAMA Cardiol, 2016, 1 (2): 147-155.

[319] Naderi SH, Bestwick JP, Wald DS. Adherence to drugs that prevent cardiovascular disease: meta-analysis on 376162 patients. Am J Med, 2012, 125 (9): 882-887, e1.

[320] Marcum ZA, Sevick MA, Handler SM. Medication nonadherence: a diagnosable and treatable medical condition. JAMA, 2013, 309 (20): 2105-2106.

[321] Castellano JM, Sanz G, Fernandez Ortiz A, et al. A polypill strategy to improve global secondary cardiovascular prevention: from concept to reality. J Am Coll Cardiol, 2014, 64 (6): 613-621.

[322] Thom S, Poulter N, Field J, et al. Effects of a fixed-dose combination strategy on adherence and risk factors in patients with or at high risk of CVD: the UMPIRE randomized clinical trial. JAMA, 2013, 310 (9): 918-929.

[323] Castellano JM, Sanz G, Peñalvo JL, et al. A polypill strategy to improve adherence: results from the FOCUS project. J Am Coll Cardiol, 2014, 64 (20): 2071-2082.

[324] Nieuwlaat R, Wilczynski N, Navarro T, et al. Interventions for enhancing medication adherence. Cochrane Database Syst Rev, 2014, 5(11): CD000011.

[325] Cahill K, Stevens S, Perera R, et al. Pharmacological interventions for smoking cessation: an overview and network meta-analysis. Cochrane Database Syst Rev, 2013, 5(5): CD009329.

[326] Hughes JR, Stead LF, Lancaster T. Antidepressants for smoking cessation. Cochrane Database Syst Rev, 2007, 1: CD000031.

[327] Cahill K, Stead LF, Lancaster T. Nicotine receptor partial agonists for smoking cessation.

Cochrane Database Syst Rev, 2012, 4: CD006103.

[328] Anderson L, Taylor RS. Cardiac rehabilitation for people with heart disease: an overview of Cochrane systematic reviews. Cochrane Database Syst Rev, 2014, 12: CD011273.

[329] Antithrombotic Trialists' (ATT) Collaboration, Baigent C, Blackwell L, et al. Aspirin in the primary and secondary prevention of vascular disease: collaborative meta-analysis of individual participant data from randomised trials. Lancet, 2009, 373 (9678): 1849-1860.

[330] CURRENT-OASIS 7 Investigators, Mehta SR, Bassand JP, et al. Dose comparisons of clopidogrel and aspirin in acute coronary syndromes. N Engl J Med, 2010, 363 (10): 930-942.

[331] Valgimigli M, Ariotti S, Costa F. Duration of dual antiplatelet therapy after drugeluting stent implantation: will we ever reach a consensus?Eur Heart J, 2015, 36 (20): 1219-1222.

[332] Costa F, Tijssen JG, Ariotti S, et al. Incremental value of the CRUSADE, ACUITY, and HAS-BLED risk scores for the prediction of hemorrhagic events after coronary stent implantation in patients undergoing long or short duration of dual antiplatelet therapy. J Am Heart Assoc, 2015, 4 (12): e002524.

[333] Bonaca MP, Bhatt DL, Cohen M, et al. Long-term use of ticagrelor in patients with prior myocardial infarction. N Engl J Med, 2015, 372 (19): 1791-1800.

[334] Mauri L, Kereiakes DJ, Yeh RW, et al. Twelve or 30 months of dual antiplatelet therapy after drug-eluting stents. N Engl J Med, 2014, 371 (23): 2155-2166.

[335] Agewall S, Cattaneo M, Collet JP, et al. Expert position paper on the use of proton pump inhibitors in patients with cardiovascular disease and antithrombotic therapy. Eur Heart J, 2013, 34 (23): 1708-1713, 1713a-1713b.

[336] Bhatt DL, Cryer BL, Contant CF, et al. Clopidogrel with or without omeprazole in coronary artery disease. N Engl J Med, 2010, 363 (20): 1909-1917.

[337] Gargiulo G, Costa F, Ariotti S, et al. Impact of proton pump inhibitors on clinical outcomes in patients treated with a 6- or 24-month dual-antiplatelet therapy duration: insights from the PROlonging Dual-antiplatelet treatment after Grading stent-induced Intimal hyperplasia study trial. Am Heart J, 2016, 174: 95-102.

[338] Mega JL, Braunwald E, Wiviott SD, et al. Rivaroxaban in patients with a recent acute coronary syndrome. N Engl J Med, 2012, 366 (1): 9-19.

[339] Palmerini T, Sangiorgi D, Valgimigli M, et al. Short-versus long-term dual antiplatelet therapy

after drug-eluting stent implantation: an individual patient data pairwise and network meta-analysis. J Am Coll Cardiol, 2015, 65 (11): 1092-1102.

[340] Palmerini T, Della Riva D, Benedetto U, et al. Three, six, or twelve months of dual antiplatelet therapy after DES implantation in patients with or without acute coronary syndromes: an individual patient data pairwise and network meta-analysis of six randomized trials and 11 473 patients. Eur Heart J, 2017, 38 (14): 1034-1043.

[341] Reeder GS, Lengyel M, Tajik AJ, et al. Mural thrombus in left ventricular aneurysm: incidence, role of angiography, and relation between anticoagulation and embolization. Mayo Clin Proc, 1981, 56 (2): 77-81.

[342] Keeley EC, Hillis LD. Left ventricular mural thrombus after acute myocardial infarction. Clinical Cardiology, 1996, 19 (2): 83-86.

[343] Turpie AG, Robinson JG, Doyle DJ, et al. Comparison of high-dose with low-dose subcutaneous heparin to prevent left ventricular mural thrombosis in patients with acute transmural anterior myocardial infarction. N Engl J Med, 1989, 320 (6): 352-357.

[344] Chen ZM, Pan HC, Chen YP, et al. Early intravenous then oral metoprolol in 45,852 patients with acute myocardial infarction: randomised placebocontrolled trial. Lancet, 2005, 366 (9497): 1622-1632.

[345] Pfisterer M, Cox JL, Granger CB, et al. Atenolol use and clinical outcomes after thrombolysis for acute myocardial infarction: the GUSTO-I experience. Global Utilization of Streptokinase and TPA (alteplase) for Occluded Coronary Arteries. J Am Coll Cardiol, 1998, 32 (3): 634-640.

[346] Chatterjee S, Chaudhuri D, Vedanthan R, et al. Early intravenous β-blockers in patients with acute coronary syndrome—a meta-analysis of randomized trials. Int J Cardiol, 2013, 168 (2): 915-921.

[347] Ibanez B, Macaya C, Sánchez-Brunete V, et al. Effect of early metoprolol on infarct size in ST-segment-elevation myocardial infarction patients undergoing primary percutaneous coronary intervention: the Effect of Metoprolol in Cardioprotection During an Acute Myocardial Infarction (METOCARD-CNIC) trial. Circulation, 2013, 128 (14): 1495-1503.

[348] Pizarro G, Fernández-Friera L, Fuster V, et al. Long-term benefit of early pre-reperfusion metoprolol administration in patients with acute myocardial infarction: results from the

METOCARD-CNIC trial (Effect of Metoprolol in Cardioprotection During an Acute Myocardial Infarction). J Am Coll Cardiol, 2014, 63 (22): 2356-2362.

[349] García-Prieto J, Villena-Gutiérrez R, Gómez M, et al. Neutrophil stunning by metoprolol reduces infarct size. Nat Commun, 2017, 8: 14780.

[350] Roolvink V, Ibáñez B, Ottervanger JP, et al. Early intravenous β-blockers in patients with ST-segment elevation myocardial infarction before primary percutaneous coronary intervention. J Am Coll Cardiol, 2016, 67 (23): 2705-2715.

[351] Halkin A, Grines CL, Cox DA, et al. Impact of intravenous β-blockade before primary angioplasty on survival in patients undergoing mechanical reperfusion therapy for acute myocardial infarction. J Am Coll Cardiol, 2004, 43 (10): 1780-1787.

[352] Harjai KJ, Stone GW, Boura J, et al. Effects of prior β-blocker therapy on clinical outcomes after primary coronary angioplasty for acute myocardial infarction. Am J Cardiol, 2003, 91 (6): 655-660.

[353] Freemantle N, Cleland J, Young P, et al. Beta blockade after myocardial infarction: systematic review and Meta regression analysis. BMJ, 1999, 318 (7200): 1730-1737.

[354] Goldberger JJ, Bonow RO, Cuffe M, et al. Effect of β-blocker dose on survival after acute myocardial infarction. J Am Coll Cardiol, 2015, 66 (13): 1431-1441.

[355] Andersson C, Shilane D, Go AS, et al. β-blocker therapy and cardiac events among patients with newly diagnosed coronary heart disease. J Am Coll Cardiol, 2014, 64 (3): 247-252.

[356] Bangalore S, Steg G, Deedwania P, et al. β-blocker use and clinical outcomes in stable outpatients with and without coronary artery disease. JAMA, 2012, 308 (13): 1340-1349.

[357] Dargie HJ. Effect of carvedilol on outcome after myocardial infarction in patients with left-ventricular dysfunction: the CAPRICORN randomised trial. Lancet, 2001, 357 (9266): 1385-1390.

[358] The Cardiac Insufficiency Bisoprolol Study II (CIBIS-II): a randomised trial. Lancet, 1999, 353 (9146): 9-13.

[359] Packer M, Coats AJ, Fowler MB, et al. Effect of carvedilol on survival in severe chronic heart failure. N Engl J Med, 2001, 344 (22): 1651-1658.

[360] Use AB. Effect of metoprolol CR/XL in chronic heart failure: Metoprolol CR/XL Randomised Intervention Trial in Congestive Heart Failure (MERIT-HF). Lancet, 1999,

353 (9169): 2001-2007.

[361] Flather MD, Shibata MC, Coats AJ, et al. Randomized trial to determine the effect of nebivolol on mortality and cardiovascular hospital admission in elderly patients with heart failure (SENIORS). Eur Heart J, 2005, 26 (3): 215-225.

[362] Bugiardini R, Cenko E, Ricci B, et al. Comparison of early versus delayed oral β blockers in acute coronary syndromes and effect on outcomes. Am J Cardiol, 2016, 117 (5): 760-767.

[363] Baigent C, Keech A, Kearney PM, et al. Efficacy and safety of cholesterol-lowering treatment: prospective meta-analysis of data from 90,056 participants in 14 randomised trials of statins. Lancet, 2005, 366 (9493): 1267-1278.

[364] Cannon CP, Braunwald E, McCabe CH, et al. Intensive versus moderate lipid lowering with statins after acute coronary syndromes. N Engl J Med, 2004, 350 (15): 1495-1504.

[365] Schwartz GG, Olsson AG, Ezekowitz MD, et al. Effects of atorvastatin on early recurrent ischemic events in acute coronary syndromes: the MIRACL study: a randomized controlled trial. JAMA, 2001, 285 (13): 1711-1718.

[366] Cholesterol Treatment Trialists' (CTT) Collaboration, Baigent C, Blackwell L, et al. Efficacy and safety of more intensive lowering of LDL cholesterol: a meta-analysis of data from 170,000 participants in 26 randomised trials. Lancet, 2010, 376 (9753): 1670-1681.

[367] Boekholdt SM, Hovingh GK, Mora S, et al. Very low levels of atherogenic lipoproteins and the risk for cardiovascular events: a meta-analysis of statin trials. J Am Coll Cardiol, 2014, 64 (5): 485-494.

[368] LaRosa JC, Grundy SM, Waters DD, et al. Intensive lipid lowering with atorvastatin in patients with stable coronary disease. N Engl J Med, 2005, 352 (14): 1425-1435.

[369] Cholesterol Treatment Trialists' (CTT) Collaboration, Fulcher J, O'Connell R, et al. Efficacy and safety of LDL-lowering therapy among men and women: meta-analysis of individual data from 174,000 participants in 27 randomised trials. Lancet, 2015, 385 (9976): 1397-1405.

[370] Shrivastava AK, Singh HV, Raizada A, et al. Serial measurement of lipid profile and inflammatory markers in patients with acute myocardial infarction. EXCLI J, 2015, 14 (14): 517-526.

[371] Pitt B, Loscalzo J, Ycas J, et al. Lipid levels after acute coronary syndromes. J Am Coll Cardiol, 2008, 51 (15): 1440-1445.

[372] Sidhu D, Naugler C. Fasting time and lipid levels in a community-based population: a cross-sectional study. Arch Intern Med, 2012, 172 (22): 1707-1710.

[373] Food and Drug Administration. FDA Drug Safety Communication: new restrictions, contraindications, and dose limitations for Zocor (simvastatin) to reduce the risk of muscle injury. http: //www.fda.gov/Drugs/DrugSafety/ucm 256581.htm, accessed July 26, 2017.

[374] Pedersen TR, Cater NB, Faergeman O, et al. Comparison of atorvastatin 80 mg/day versus simvastatin 20 to 40 mg/day on frequency of cardiovascular events late (five years) after acute myocardial infarction (from the Incremental Decrease in End Points through Aggressive Lipid Lowering [IDEAL] trial). Am J Cardiol, 2010, 106 (3): 354-359.

[375] Tikkanen MJ, Szarek M, Fayyad R, et al. Total cardiovascular disease burden: comparing intensive with moderate statin therapy insights from the IDEAL (Incremental Decrease in End Points Through Aggressive Lipid Lowering) trial. J Am Coll Cardiol, 2009, 54 (25): 2353-2357.

[376] Cannon CP, Blazing MA, Giugliano RP, et al. Ezetimibe added to statin therapy after acute coronary syndromes. N Engl J Med, 2015, 372 (25): 2387-2397.

[377] Li C, Lin L, Zhang W, et al. Efficiency and safety of proprotein convertase subtilisin/kexin 9 monoclonal antibody on hypercholesterolemia: a meta-analysis of 20 randomized controlled trials. J Am Heart Assoc, 2015, 4 (6): e001937.

[378] Zhang XL, Zhu QQ, Zhu L, et al. Safety and efficacy of anti-PCSK9 antibodies: a meta-analysis of 25 randomized, controlled trials. BMC Med, 2015, 13 (1): 123.

[379] Sabatine MS, Giugliano RP, Wiviott SD, et al. Efficacy and safety of evolocumab in reducing lipids and cardiovascular events. N Engl J Med, 2015, 372 (16): 1500-1509.

[380] Robinson JG, Farnier M, Krempf M, et al. Efficacy and safety of alirocumab in reducing lipids and cardiovascular events. N Engl J Med, 2015, 372 (16): 1489-1499.

[381] Navarese EP, Kolodziejczak M, Schulze V, et al. Effects of proprotein convertase subtilisin/kexin type 9 antibodies in adults with hypercholesterolemia: a systematic review and meta-analysis. Ann Intern Med, 2015, 163 (1): 40-51.

[382] Sabatine MS, Giugliano RP, Keech AC, et al. Evolocumab and clinical outcomes in patients with cardiovascular disease. N Engl J Med, 2017, 376 (18): 1713-1722.

[383] ISIS-4 (Fourth International Study of Infarct Survival) Collaborative Group. ISIS- 4: a

randomised factorial trial assessing early oral captopril, oral mononitrate, and intravenous magnesium sulphate in 58,050 patients with suspected acute myocardial infarction. Lancet, 1995, 345 (8951): 669-685.

[384] Yusuf S, Held P, Furberg C. Update of effects of calcium antagonists in myocardial infarction or angina in light of the second Danish Verapamil Infarction Trial (DAVIT- II) and other recent studies. Am J Cardiol, 1991, 67 (15): 1295-1297.

[385] Held PH, Yusuf S, Furberg CD. Calcium channel blockers in acute myocardial infarction and unstable angina: an overview. BMJ, 1989, 299 (6709): 1187-1192.

[386] . Effect of verapamil on mortality and major events after acute myocardial infarction (the Danish Verapamil Infarction Trial II–DAVIT II). Am J Cardiol, 1990, 66 (10): 779-785.

[387] Furberg CD, Psaty BM, Meyer JV. Nifedipine. Dose-related increase in mortality in patients with coronary heart disease. Circulation, 1995, 92 (5): 1326-1331.

[388] Poole-Wilson PA, Lubsen J, Kirwan BA, et al. Effect of long-acting nifedipine on mortality and cardiovascular morbidity in patients with stable angina requiring treatment (ACTION trial): randomised controlled trial. Lancet, 2004, 364 (9437): 849-857.

[389] Pfeffer MA, Greaves SC, Arnold JM, et al. Early versus delayed angiotensin-converting enzyme inhibition therapy in acute myocardial infarction. The healing and early afterload reducing therapy trial. Circulation, 1997, 95 (12): 2643-2651.

[390] Køber L, Torp-Pedersen C, Carlsen JE, et al. A clinical trial of the angiotensin-converting-enzyme inhibitor trandolapril in patients with left ventricular dysfunction after myocardial infarction. Trandolapril Cardiac Evaluation (TRACE) Study Group. N Engl J Med, 1995, 333 (25): 1670-1676.

[391] Ball SG, Hall AS, Murray GD. ACE inhibition, atherosclerosis and myocardial infarction—the AIRE Study in practice. Acute Infarction Ramipril Efficacy Study. Eur Heart J, 1994, 15 (Suppl B): 20-25, discussion 26-30.

[392] Pfeffer MA, Braunwald E, Moyé LA, et al. Effect of captopril on mortality and morbidity in patients with left ventricular dysfunction after myocardial infarction. Results of the survival and ventricular enlargement trial. The SAVE Investigators. N Engl J Med, 1992, 327 (10): 669-677.

[393] ACE Inhibitor Myocardial Infarction Collaborative Group. Indications for ACE inhibitors

in the early treatment of acute myocardial infarction: systematic overview of individual data from 100,000 patients in randomized trials. Circulation, 1998, 97 (22): 2202-2212.

[394] Fox KM, EURopean trial On reduction of cardiac events with Perindopril in stable coronary Artery disease Investigators. Efficacy of perindopril in reduction of cardiovascular events among patients with stable coronary artery disease: randomised, double-blind, placebo-controlled, multicentre trial (the EUROPA study). Lancet, 2003, 362 (9386): 782-788.

[395] Heart Outcomes Prevention Evaluation Study Investigators, Yusuf S, Sleight P, et al. Effects of an angiotensin-converting-enzyme inhibitor, ramipril, on cardiovascular events in high-risk patients. N Engl J Med, 2000, 342 (3): 145-153.

[396] Pfeffer MA, McMurray JJ, Velazquez EJ, et al. Valsartan, captopril, or both in myocardial infarction complicated by heart failure, left ventricular dysfunction, or both. N Engl J Med, 2003, 349 (20): 1893-1906.

[397] Pitt B, Remme W, Zannad F, et al. Eplerenone, a selective aldosterone blocker, in patients with left ventricular dysfunction after myocardial infarction. N Engl J Med, 2003, 348 (14): 1309-1321.

[398] Pitt B, Zannad F, Remme WJ, et al. The effect of spironolactone on morbidity and mortality in patients with severe heart failure. Randomized Aldactone Evaluation Study Investigators. N Engl J Med, 1999, 341 (10): 709-717.

[399] Zannad F, McMurray JJ, Krum H, et al. Eplerenone in patients with systolic heart failure and mild symptoms. N Engl J Med, 2011, 364 (1): 11-21.

[400] Girerd N, Collier T, Pocock S, et al. Clinical benefits of eplerenone in patients with systolic heart failure and mild symptoms when initiated shortly after hospital discharge: analysis from the EMPHASIS-HF trial. Eur Heart J, 2015, 36 (34): 2310-2317.

[401] Montalescot G, Pitt B, Lopez de Sa E, et al. Early eplerenone treatment in patients with acute ST-elevation myocardial infarction without heart failure: the Randomized Double-Blind Reminder Study. Eur Heart J, 2014, 35 (34): 2295-2302.

[402] Beygui F, Cayla G, Roule V, et al. Early aldosterone blockade in acute myocardial infarction: the ALBATROSS Randomized Clinical Trial. J Am Coll Cardiol, 2016, 67 (16): 1917-1927.

[403] García-Ruiz JM, Fernández-Jiménez R, García-Alvarez A, et al. Impact of the timing of metoprolol administration during STEMI on infarct size and ventricular function. J Am Coll

Cardiol, 2016, 67 (18): 2093-2104.

[404] Bangalore S, Makani H, Radford M, et al. Clinical outcomes with β-blockers for myocardial infarction: a meta-analysis of randomized trials. Am J Med, 2014, 127 (10): 939-953.

[405] Huang BT, Huang FY, Zuo ZL, et al. Meta-analysis of relation between oral β-blocker therapy and outcomes in patients with acute myocardial infarction who underwent percutaneous coronary intervention. Am J Cardiol, 2015, 115 (11): 1529-1538.

[406] Catapano AL, Graham I, De Backer G, et al. 2016 ESC/EAS Guidelines for the Management of Dyslipidaemias: the Task Force for the Management of Dyslipidaemias of the European Society of Cardiology (ESC) and European Atherosclerosis Society (EAS) Developed with the special contribution of the European Assocciation for Cardiovascular Prevention & Rehabilitation (EACPR). Atherosclerosis, 2016, 253: 281-344.

[407] Dickstein K, Kjekshus J, Optimaal Steering Committee of the OPTIMAAL Study Group. Effects of losartan and captopril on mortality and morbidity in high-risk patients after acute myocardial infarction: the OPTIMAAL randomised trial. Optimal Trial in Myocardial Infarction with Angiotensin Ⅱ Antagonist Losartan. Lancet, 2002, 360 (9335): 752-760.

[408] Iakobishvili Z, Cohen E, Garty M, et al. Use of intravenous morphine for acute decompensated heart failure in patients with and without acute coronary syndromes. Acute Card Care, 2011, 13 (2): 76-80.

[409] Peacock WF, Hollander JE, Diercks DB, et al. Morphine and outcomes in acute decompensated heart failure: an ADHERE analysis. Emerg Med J, 2008, 25 (4): 205-209.

[410] Weng CL, Zhao YT, Liu QH, et al. Meta-analysis: noninvasive ventilation in acute cardiogenic pulmonary edema. Ann Intern Med, 2010, 152 (9): 590-600.

[411] Vital FM, Ladeira MT, Atallah AN. Non-invasive positive pressure ventilation (CPAP or bilevel NPPV) for cardiogenic pulmonary oedema. Cochrane Database Syst Rev, 2013, 5 (5): CD005351.

[412] McAlister FA, Stewart S, Ferrua S, et al. Multidisciplinary strategies for the management of heart failure patients at high risk for admission: a systematic review of randomized trials. J Am Coll Cardiol, 2004, 44 (4): 810-819.

[413] The Acute Infarction Ramipril Efficacy (AIRE) Study Investigators. Effect of ramipril on mortality and morbidity of survivors of acute myocardial infarction with clinical evidence of

heart failure. Lancet, 1993, 342 (8875): 821-828.

[414] Hjalmarson A, Goldstein S, Fagerberg B, et al. Effects of controlled-release metoprolol on total mortality, hospitalizations, and well-being in patients with heart failure: the Metoprolol CR/XL Randomized Intervention Trial in congestive heart failure (MERIT-HF). MERIT-HF Study Group. JAMA, 2000, 283 (10): 1295-1302.

[415] Packer M, Bristow MR, Cohn JN, et al. The effect of carvedilol on morbidity and mortality in patients with chronic heart failure. U.S. Carvedilol Heart Failure Study Group. N Engl J Med, 1996, 334 (21): 1349-1355.

[416] Packer M, Fowler MB, Roecker EB, et al. Effect of carvedilol on the morbidity of patients with severe chronic heart failure: results of the carvedilol prospective randomized cumulative survival (COPERNICUS) study. Circulation, 2002, 106 (17): 2194-2199.

[417] Gray AJ, Goodacre S, Newby DE, et al. A multicentre randomised controlled trial of the use of continuous positive airway pressure and non-invasive positive pressure ventilation in the early treatment of patients presenting to the emergency department with severe acute cardiogenic pulmonary oedema: the 3CPO trial. Health Technol Assess, 2009, 13 (33): 1-106.

[418] Park M, Sangean MC, Volpe Mde S, et al. Randomized, prospective trial of oxygen, continuous positive airway pressure, and bilevel positive airway pressure by face mask in acute cardiogenic pulmonary edema. Crit Care Med, 2004, 32 (12): 2407-2415.

[419] Gray A, Goodacre S, Newby DE, et al. Noninvasive ventilation in acute cardiogenic pulmonary edema. N Engl J Med, 2008, 359 (2): 142-151.

[420] Harjola VP, Mebazaa A, Celutkiene J, et al. Contemporary management of acute right ventricular failure: a statement from the Heart Failure Association and the Working Group on Pulmonary Circulation and Right Ventricular Function of the European Society of Cardiology. Eur J Heart Fail, 2016, 18 (3): 226-241.

[421] Goldberg RJ, Spencer FA, Gore JM, et al. Thirty-year trends (1975 to 2005) in the magnitude of, management of, and hospital death rates associated with cardiogenic shock in patients with acute myocardial infarction: a population-based perspective. Circulation, 2009, 119 (9): 1211-1219.

[422] Picard MH, Davidoff R, Sleeper LA, et al. Echocardiographic predictors of survival and response to early revascularization in cardiogenic shock. Circulation, 2003, 107 (2): 279-284.

[423] Engstrom AE, Vis MM, Bouma BJ, et al. Right ventricular dysfunction is an independent predictor for mortality in ST-elevation myocardial infarction patients presenting with cardiogenic shock on admission. Eur J Heart Fail, 2010, 12 (3): 276-282.

[424] Jeger RV, Lowe AM, Buller CE, et al. Hemodynamic parameters are prognostically important in cardiogenic shock but similar following early revascularization or initial medical stabilization: a report from the SHOCK trial. Chest, 2007, 132 (6): 1794-1803.

[425] TRIUMPH Investigators, Alexander JH, Reynolds HR, et al. Effect of tilarginine acetate in patients with acute myocardial infarction and cardiogenic shock: the TRIUMPH randomized controlled trial. JAMA, 2007, 297 (15): 1657-1666.

[426] Lancellotti P, Price S, Edvardsen T, et al. The use of echocardiography in acute cardiovascular care: recommendations of the European Association of Cardiovascular Imaging and the Acute Cardiovascular Care Association. Eur Heart J Acute Cardiovasc Care, 2015, 4 (1): 3-5.

[427] Hussain F, Philipp RK, Ducas RA, et al. The ability to achieve complete revascularization is associated with improved in-hospital survival in cardiogenic shock due to myocardial infarction: Manitoba cardiogenic SHOCK Registry investigators. Catheter Cardiovasc Interv, 2011, 78 (4): 540-548.

[428] De Backer D, Biston P, Devriendt J, et al. Comparison of dopamine and norepinephrine in the treatment of shock. N Engl J Med, 2010, 362 (9): 779-789.

[429] Ouweneel DM, Eriksen E, Sjauw KD, et al. Percutaneous mechanical circulatory support versus intra-aortic balloon pump in cardiogenic shock after acute myocardial infarction. J Am Coll Cardiol, 2017, 69 (3): 278-287.

[430] Cheng JM, den Uil CA, Hoeks SE, et al. Percutaneous left ventricular assist devices vs. intra-aortic balloon pump counterpulsation for treatment of cardiogenic shock: a meta-analysis of controlled trials. Eur Heart J, 2009, 30 (17): 2102-2108.

[431] Starling RC, Naka Y, Boyle AJ, et al. Results of the post-US Food and Drug Administrationapproval study with a continuous flow left ventricular assist device as a bridge to heart transplantation. A prospective study using the INTERMACS (Interagency Registry for Mechanically Assisted Circulatory Support). J Am Coll Cardiol, 2011, 57 (19): 1890-1898.

[432] Sheu JJ, Tsai TH, Lee FY, et al. Early extracorporeal membrane oxygenator-assisted primary

percutaneous coronary intervention improved 30-day clinical outcomes in patients with ST-segment elevation myocardial infarction complicated with profound cardiogenic shock. Crit Care Med, 2010, 38 (9): 1810-1817.

[433] Shah MR, Hasselblad V, Stevenson LW, et al. Impact of the pulmonary artery catheter in critically ill patients: meta-analysis of randomized clinical trials. JAMA, 2005, 294 (13): 1664-1670.

[434] Bart BA, Goldsmith SR, Lee KL, et al. Ultrafiltration in decompensated heart failure with cardiorenal syndrome. N Engl J Med, 2012, 367 (24): 2296-2304.

[435] Costanzo MR, Guglin ME, Saltzberg MT, et al. Ultrafiltration versus intravenous diuretics for patients hospitalized for acute decompensated heart failure. J Am Coll Cardiol, 2007, 49 (6): 675-683.

[436] Costanzo MR, Saltzberg MT, Jessup M, et al. Ultrafiltration is associated with fewer rehospitalizations than continuous diuretic infusion in patients with decompensated heart failure: results from UNLOAD. J Card Fail, 2010, 16 (4): 277-284.

[437] Buerke M, Prondzinsky R, Lemm H, et al. Intra-aortic balloon counterpulsation in the treatment of infarction-related cardiogenic shock—review of the current evidence. Artif Organs, 2012, 36 (6): 505-511.

[438] Gorenek B, Blomström Lundqvist C, Brugada Terradellas J, et al. Cardiac arrhythmias in acute coronary syndromes: position paper from the joint EHRA, ACCA, and EAPCI task force. Europace, 2014, 16 (11): 1655-1673.

[439] Piccini JP, Schulte PJ, Pieper KS, et al. Antiarrhythmic drug therapy for sustained ventricular arrhythmias complicating acute myocardial infarction. Crit Care Med, 2011, 39 (1): 78-83.

[440] Piers SR, Wijnmaalen AP, Borleffs CJ, et al. Early reperfusion therapy affects inducibility, cycle length, and occurrence of ventricular tachycardia late after myocardial infarction. Circ Arrhythm Electrophysiol, 2011, 4 (2): 195-201.

[441] Nalliah CJ, Zaman S, Narayan A, et al. Coronary artery reperfusion for ST elevation myocardial infarction is associated with shorter cycle length ventricular tachycardia and fewer spontaneous arrhythmias. Europace, 2014, 16 (7): 1053-1060.

[442] Liang JJ, Fender EA, Cha YM, et al. Long-term outcomes in survivors of early ventricular arrhythmias after acute ST-elevation and non-ST-elevation myocardial infarction treated with

percutaneous coronary intervention. Am J Cardiol, 2016, 117 (5): 709-713.

[443] Danchin N, Fauchier L, Marijon E, et al. Impact of early statin therapy on development of atrial fibrillation at the acute stage of myocardial infarction: data from the FAST-MI register. Heart, 2010, 96 (22): 1809-1814.

[444] Schmitt J, Duray G, Gersh BJ, et al. Atrial fibrillation in acute myocardial infarction: a systematic review of the incidence, clinical features and prognostic implications. Eur Heart J, 2009, 30 (9): 1038-1045.

[445] Batra G, Svennblad B, Held C, et al. All types of atrial fibrillation in the setting of myocardial infarction are associated with impaired outcome. Heart, 2016, 102 (12): 926-933.

[446] Nilsson KR Jr, Al-Khatib SM, Zhou Y, et al. Atrial fibrillation management strategies and early mortality after myocardial infarction: results from the Valsartan in Acute Myocardial Infarction (VALIANT) Trial. Heart, 2010, 96 (11): 838-842.

[447] Jabre P, Jouven X, Adnet F, et al. Atrial fibrillation and death after myocardial infarction: a community study. Circulation, 2011, 123 (19): 2094-2100.

[448] Siu CW, Jim MH, Ho HH, et al. Transient atrial fibrillation complicating acute inferior myocardial infarction: implications for future risk of ischemic stroke. Chest, 2007, 132 (1): 44-49.

[449] Segal JB, McNamara RL, Miller MR, et al. The evidence regarding the drugs used for ventricular rate control. J Fam Pract, 2000, 49 (1): 47-59.

[450] Hou ZY, Chang MS, Chen CY, et al. Acute treatment of recent-onset atrial fibrillation and flutter with a tailored dosing regimen of intravenous amiodarone. A randomized, digoxin-controlled study. Eur Heart J, 1995, 16 (4): 521-528.

[451] Metawee M, Charnigo R, Morales G, et al. Digoxin and short term mortality after acute STEMI: results from the MAGIC trial. Int J Cardiol, 2016, 218: 176-180.

[452] Jordaens L, Trouerbach J, Calle P, et al. Conversion of atrial fibrillation to sinus rhythm and rate control by digoxin in comparison to placebo. Eur Heart J, 1997, 18 (4): 643-648.

[453] Thomas SP, Guy D, Wallace E, et al. Rapid loading of sotalol or amiodarone for management of recent onset symptomatic atrial fibrillation: a randomized, digoxin-controlled trial. Am Heart J, 2004, 147 (1): E3.

[454] Piccini JP, Hranitzky PM, Kilaru R, et al. Relation of mortality to failure to prescribe beta

blockers acutely in patients with sustained ventricular tachycardia and ventricular fibrillation following acute myocardial infarction (from the VALsartan In Acute myocardial iNfarcTion trial [VALIANT] Registry). Am J Cardiol, 2008, 102 (11): 1427-1432.

[455] Zafari AM, Zarter SK, Heggen V, et al. A program encouraging early defibrillation results in improved in-hospital resuscitation efficacy. J Am Coll Cardiol, 2004, 44 (4): 846-852.

[456] Wolfe CL, Nibley C, Bhandari A, et al. Polymorphous ventricular tachycardia associated with acute myocardial infarction. Circulation, 1991, 84 (4): 1543-1551.

[457] Mehta RH, Yu J, Piccini JP, et al. Prognostic significance of postprocedural sustained ventricular tachycardia or fibrillation in patients undergoing primary percutaneous coronary intervention (from the HORIZONS-AMI Trial). Am J Cardiol, 2012, 109 (6): 805-812.

[458] Masuda M, Nakatani D, Hikoso S, et al. Clinical impact of ventricular tachycardia and/or fibrillation during the acute phase of acute myocardial infarction on in-hospital and 5-year mortality rates in the percutaneous coronary intervention era. Circ J, 2016, 80 (7): 1539-1547.

[459] Haissaguerre M, Vigmond E, Stuyvers B, et al. Ventricular arrhythmias and the His-Purkinje system. Nat Rev Cardiol, 2016, 13 (3): 155-166.

[460] Enjoji Y, Mizobuchi M, Muranishi H, et al. Catheter ablation of fatal ventricular tachyarrhythmias storm in acute coronary syndrome—role of Purkinje fiber network. J Interv Card Electrophysiol, 2009, 26 (3): 207-215.

[461] Peichl P, Cihak R, Kozeluhova M, et al. Catheter ablation of arrhythmic storm triggered by monomorphic ectopic beats in patients with coronary artery disease. J Interv Card Electrophysiol, 2010, 27 (1): 51-59.

[462] Nademanee K, Taylor R, Bailey WE, et al. Treating electrical storm: sympathetic blockade versus advanced cardiac life support-guided therapy. Circulation, 2000, 102 (7): 742-747.

[463] Miwa Y, Ikeda T, Mera H, et al. Effects of landiolol, an ultra-short-acting beta1-selective blocker, on electrical storm refractory to class III antiarrhythmic drugs. Circ J, 2010, 74 (5): 856-863.

[464] Hine LK, Laird N, Hewitt P, et al. Meta-analytic evidence against prophylactic use of lidocaine in acute myocardial infarction. Arch Intern Med, 1989, 149 (12): 2694-2698.

[465] Huikuri HV, Castellanos A, Myerburg RJ. Sudden death due to cardiac arrhythmias. N Engl J Med, 2001, 345 (20): 1473-1482.

[466] Moss AJ, Zareba W, Hall WJ, et al. Prophylactic implantation of a defibrillator in patients with myocardial infarction and reduced ejection fraction. N Engl J Med, 2002, 346 (12): 877-883.

[467] Bardy GH, Lee KL, Mark DB, et al. Amiodarone or an implantable cardioverter-defibrillator for congestive heart failure. N Engl J Med, 2005, 352 (3): 225-237.

[468] Chen A, Ashburn MA. Cardiac effects of opioid therapy. Pain Med, 2015, 16 (Suppl 1): S27-S31.

[469] Brignole M, Auricchio A, Baron-Esquivias G, et al. 2013 ESC Guidelines on cardiac pacing and cardiac resynchronization therapy. The Task Force on cardiac pacing and resynchronization therapy of the European Society of Cardiology (ESC). Developed in collaboration with the European Heart Rhythm Association (EHRA). Eur Heart J, 2013, 34 (29): 2281-2329.

[470] Caforio AL, Pankuweit S, Arbustini E, et al. Current state of knowledge on aetiology, diagnosis, management, and therapy of myocarditis: a position statement of the European Society of Cardiology Working Group on Myocardial and Pericardial Diseases. Eur Heart J, 2013, 34 (33): 2636-2648, 2648a-2648d.

[471] Emrich T, Emrich K, Abegunewardene N, et al. Cardiac MR enables diagnosis in 90% of patients with acute chest pain, elevated biomarkers and unobstructed coronary arteries. Br J Radiol, 2015, 88 (1049): 20150025.

[472] Pathik B, Raman B, Mohd Amin NH, et al. Troponin-positive chest pain with unobstructed coronary arteries: incremental diagnostic value of cardiovascular magnetic resonance imaging. Eur Heart J Cardiovasc Imaging, 2016, 17 (10): 1146-1152.

[473] Dastidar AG, Rodrigues JC, Johnson TW, et al. Myocardial Infarction with nonobstructed coronary arteries: impact of CMR early after presentation. JACC Cardiovasc Imaging, 2017, 10 (10 Pt A): 1204-1206.

[474] Fox KA, Goodman SG, Klein W, et al. Management of acute coronary syndromes. Variations in practice and outcome; findings from the Global Registry of Acute Coronary Events (GRACE). Eur Heart J, 2002, 23 (15): 1177-1189.

[475] Lenfant C. Shattuck lecture--clinical research to clinical practice--lost in translation?N Engl J Med, 2003, 349 (9): 868-874.

[476] Schiele F, Gale CP, Bonnefoy E, et al. Quality indicators for acute myocardial infarction: a position paper of the Acute Cardiovascular Care Association. Eur Heart J Acute Cardiovasc Care, 2017, 6 (1): 34-59.

[477] Ford I, Norrie J. Pragmatic trials. N Engl J Med, 2016, 375 (5): 454-463.

[478] Rossini R, Angiolillo DJ, Musumeci G, et al. Aspirin desensitization in patients undergoing percutaneous coronary interventions with stent implantation. Am J Cardiol, 2008, 101 (6): 786-789.

[479] CAPRIE Steering Committee. A randomised, blinded, trial of clopidogrel versus aspirin in patients at risk of ischaemic events (CAPRIE). CAPRIE Steering Committee. Lancet, 1996, 348 (9038): 1329-1339.

[480] Navarese EP, Andreotti F, Schulze V, et al. Optimal duration of dual antiplatelet therapy after percutaneous coronary intervention with drug eluting stents: meta-analysis of randomised controlled trials. BMJ, 2015, 350: h1618.

[481] Valgimigli M, Campo G, Monti M, et al. Short-versus long-term duration of dualantiplatelet therapy after coronary stenting: a randomized multicenter trial. Circulation, 2012, 125 (16): 2015-2026.

[482] Morrow DA, Braunwald E, Bonaca MP, et al. Vorapaxar in the secondary prevention of atherothrombotic events. N Engl J Med, 2012, 366 (15): 1404-1413.

[483] Ng VG, Lansky AJ, Meller S, et al. The prognostic importance of left ventricular function in patients with ST-segment elevation myocardial infarction: the HORIZONS-AMI trial. Eur Heart J Acute Cardiovasc Care, 2014, 3 (1): 67-77.

[484] Sutton NR, Li S, Thomas L, et al. The association of left ventricular ejection fraction with clinical outcomes after myocardial infarction: findings from the Acute Coronary Treatment and Intervention Outcomes Network (ACTION) Registry-Get with the Guidelines (GWTG) Medicare-linked database. Am Heart J, 2016, 178: 65-73.

[485] Jones RH, Velazquez EJ, Michler RE, et al. Coronary bypass surgery with or without surgical ventricular reconstruction. N Engl J Med, 2009, 360 (17): 1705-1717.

[486] Di Donato M, Castelvecchio S, Brankovic J, et al. Effectiveness of surgical ventricular restoration in patients with dilated ischemic cardiomyopathy and unrepaired mild mitral regurgitation. J Thorac Cardiovasc Surg, 2007, 134 (6): 1548-1553.

[487] Weinsaft JW, Kim J, Medicherla CB, et al. Echocardiographic algorithm for post-myocardial infarction lv thrombus: a gatekeeper for thrombus evaluation by delayed enhancement CMR. JACC Cardiovasc Imaging, 2016, 9 (5): 505-515.

[488] Pöss J, Desch S, Eitel C, et al. Left ventricular thrombus formation after ST-segment-elevation myocardial infarction: insights from a cardiac magnetic resonance multicenter study. Circ Cardiovasc Imaging, 2015, 8 (10): e003417.

[489] Solheim S, Seljeflot I, Lunde K, et al. Frequency of left ventricular thrombus in patients with anterior wall acute myocardial infarction treated with percutaneous coronary intervention and dual antiplatelet therapy. Am J Cardiol, 2010, 106 (9): 1197-1200.

[490] Meurin P, Brandao Carreira V, Dumaine R, et al. Incidence, diagnostic methods, and evolution of left ventricular thrombus in patients with anterior myocardial infarction and low left ventricular ejection fraction: a prospective multicenter study. Am Heart J, 2015, 170 (2): 256-262.

[491] Delewi R, Zijlstra F, Piek JJ. Left ventricular thrombus formation after acute myocardial infarction. Heart, 2012, 98 (23): 1743-1749.

[492] Lip GY, Windecker S, Huber K, et al. Management of antithrombotic therapy in atrial fibrillation patients presenting with acute coronary syndrome and/or undergoing percutaneous coronary or valve interventions: a joint consensus document of the European Society of Cardiology Working Group on Thrombosis, European Heart Rhythm Association (EHRA) , European Association of Percutaneous Cardiovascular Interventions (EAPCI) and European Association of Acute Cardiac Care (ACCA) endorsed by the Heart Rhythm Society (HRS) and Asia-Pacific Heart Rhythm Society (APHRS). Eur Heart J, 2014, 35 (45): 3155-3179.

[493] Vahanian A, Iung B. Severe secondary mitral regurgitation and left ventricular dysfunction: a'deadly combination'against which the fight is not over!Eur Heart J, 2015, 36 (40): 2742-2744.

[494] Abate E, Hoogslag GE, Al Amri I, et al. Time course, predictors, and prognostic implications of significant mitral regurgitation after ST-segment elevation myocardial infarction. Am Heart J, 2016, 178: 115-125.

[495] Ray S. The echocardiographic assessment of functional mitral regurgitation. Eur J Echocardiogr, 2010, 11 (10): i11-i17.

[496] Alajaji WA, Akl EA, Farha A, et al. Surgical versus medical management of patients with acute ischemic mitral regurgitation: a systematic review. BMC Res Notes, 2015, 8 (1): 712.

[497] Lorusso R, Gelsomino S, De Cicco G, et al. Mitral valve surgery in emergency for severe acute regurgitation: analysis of postoperative results from a multicentre study. Eur J Cardiothorac Surg, 2008, 33 (4): 573-582.

[498] Masci PG, Francone M, Desmet W, et al. Right ventricular ischemic injury in patients with acute ST-segment elevation myocardial infarction: characterization with cardiovascular magnetic resonance. Circulation, 2010, 122 (14): 1405-1412.

[499] Mehta SR, Eikelboom JW, Natarajan MK, et al. Impact of right ventricular involvement on mortality and morbidity in patients with inferior myocardial infarction. J Am Coll Cardiol, 2001, 37 (1): 37-43.

[500] Bowers TR, O'Neill WW, Grines C, et al. Effect of reperfusion on biventricular function and survival after right ventricular infarction. N Engl J Med, 1998, 338 (14): 933-940.

[501] Lupi-Herrera E, González-Pacheco H, Juárez-Herrera U, et al. Primary reperfusion in acute right ventricular infarction: an observational study. World J Cardiol, 2014, 6 (1): 14-22.

[502] Kinn JW, Ajluni SC, Samyn JG, et al. Rapid hemodynamic improvement after reperfusion during right ventricular infarction. J Am Coll Cardiol, 1995, 26 (5): 1230-1234.

[503] Velagaleti RS, Pencina MJ, Murabito JM, et al. Long-term trends in the incidence of heart failure after myocardial infarction. Circulation, 2008, 118 (20): 2057-2062.

[504] Desta L, Jernberg T, Löfman I, et al. Incidence, temporal trends, and prognostic impact of heart failure complicating acute myocardial infarction. The SWEDEHEART Registry (Swedish Web-System for Enhancement and Development of Evidence-Based Care in Heart Disease Evaluated According to Recommended Therapies): a study of 199, 851 patients admitted with index acute myocardial infarctions, 1996 to 2008. JACC Heart Fail, 2015, 3 (3): 234-242.

[505] Lancellotti P, Price S, Edvardsen T, et al. The use of echocardiography in acute cardiovascular care: Recommendations of the European Association of Cardiovascular Imaging and the Acute Cardiovascular Care Association. Eur Heart J Acute Cardiovasc Care, 2014.

[506] Cheng JM, Helming AM, van Vark LC, et al. A simple risk chart for initial risk assessment of 30-day mortality in patients with cardiogenic shock from ST-elevation myocardial infarction.

Eur Heart J Acute Cardiovasc Care, 2016, 5 (2): 101-107.

[507]   Haddadin S, Milano AD, Faggian G, et al. Surgical treatment of postinfarction left ventricular free wall rupture. J Card Surg, 2009, 24 (6): 624-631.

[508]   Figueras J, Alcalde O, Barrabés JA, et al. Changes in hospital mortality rates in 425 patients with acute ST-elevation myocardial infarction and cardiac rupture over a 30-year period. Circulation, 2008, 118 (25): 2783-2789.

[509]   Porto AG, McAlindon E, Ascione R, et al. Magnetic resonance imaging-based management of silent cardiac rupture. J Thorac Cardiovasc Surg, 2015, 149 (3): e31-e33.

[510]   Karamitsos TD, Ferreira V, Banerjee R, et al. Contained left ventricular rupture after acute myocardial infarction revealed by cardiovascular magnetic resonance imaging. Circulation, 2012, 125 (18): 2278-2280.

[511]   Topaz O, Taylor AL. Interventricular septal rupture complicating acute myocardial infarction: from pathophysiologic features to the role of invasive and noninvasive diagnostic modalities in current management. Am J Med, 1992, 93 (6): 683-688.

[512]   Lemery R, Smith HC, Giuliani ER, et al. Prognosis in rupture of the ventricular septum after acute myocardial infarction and role of early surgical intervention. Am J Cardiol, 1992, 70 (2): 147-151.

[513]   Calvert PA, Cockburn J, Wynne D, et al. Percutaneous closure of postinfarction ventricular septal defect: in-hospital outcomes and long-term follow-up of UK experience. Circulation, 2014, 129 (23): 2395-2402.

[514]   Thompson CR, Buller CE, Sleeper LA, et al. Cardiogenic shock due to acute severe mitral regurgitation complicating acute myocardial infarction: a report from the SHOCK Trial Registry. SHould we use emergently revascularize Occluded Coronaries in cardiogenic shocK?J Am Coll Cardiol, 2000, 36 (3 Suppl A): 1104-1109.

[515]   Bajaj A, Sethi A, Rathor P, et al. Acute complications of myocardial infarction in the current era: diagnosis and management. J Investig Med, 2015, 63 (7): 844-855.

[516]   Fasol R, Lakew F, Wetter S. Mitral repair in patients with a ruptured papillary muscle. Am Heart J, 2000, 139 (3): 549-554.

[517]   Imazio M, Negro A, Belli R, et al. Frequency and prognostic significance of pericarditis following acute myocardial infarction treated by primary percutaneous coronary intervention.

Am J Cardiol, 2009, 103 (11): 1525-1529.

[518] Adler Y, Charron P, Imazio M, et al. 2015 ESC Guidelines for the diagnosis and management of pericardial diseases: the Task Force for the Diagnosis and Management of Pericardial Diseases of the European Society of Cardiology (ESC). Endorsed by: the European Association for Cardio-Thoracic Surgery (EACTS). Eur Heart J, 2015, 36 (42): 2921-2964.

[519] Bebb O, Hall M, Fox KAA, et al. Performance of hospitals according to the ESC ACCA quality indicators and 30- day mortality for acute myocardial infarction: national cohort study using the United Kingdom Myocardial Ischaemia National Audit Project (MINAP) register. Eur Heart J, 2017, 38 (13): 974-982.

[520] Simms AD, Batin PD, Weston CF, et al. An evaluation of composite indicators of hospital acute myocardial infarction care: a study of 136, 392 patients from the Myocardial Ischaemia National Audit Project. Int J Cardiol, 2013, 170 (1): 81-87.